BARBARA E
& DEIRDRE ENGLISH

Complaints and Disorders

The Sexual Politics of Sickness

SECOND EDITION

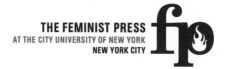

THE FEMINIST PRESS
AT THE CITY UNIVERSITY OF NEW YORK
NEW YORK CITY

Published in 2011 by the Feminist Press
at the City University of New York
The Graduate Center
365 Fifth Avenue, Suite 5406
New York, NY 10016

feministpress.org

First Feminist Press edition published 1973
Second edition with new introduction published July 2011
Third printing, November 2018

Cover design by John Yates/Stealworks
Text design by Drew Stevens

Library of Congress Cataloging-in-Publication Data

Ehrenreich, Barbara.
 Complaints and disorders : the sexual politics of sickness / Barbara Ehrenreich
& Deirdre English. — 2nd ed.
   p. ; cm. — (Contemporary classics)
 ISBN 978-1-55861-695-0 (pbk.)
1. Women—Health and hygiene—Sociological aspects. I. English, Deirdre.
II. Title. III. Series: Contemporary classics (Feminist Press)
 [DNLM: 1. Women's Health—history—United States. 2. History, 19th
Century—United States. 3. History, 20th Century—United States. 4. Prejudice—
United States. 5. Social Conditions—history—United States. 6. Socioeconomic
Factors—history—United States. 7. Women's Rights—history—United States.
WA 11 AA1]
 RG121.E43 2011
 362.1082—dc22

                                                              2011011650

Contents

Introduction

SUSAN FALUDI

A STORY FROM THE '70s: A YOUNG WOMAN GOES TO
see a gynecologist. She is seeking contraceptives. The
doctor questions why she needs them. She thinks this
is patronizing and none of his business. "I'm going
to college," is all she will say. He frowns, not used to
obstinate behavior from female patients. Finally, seeing she is not to be dissuaded, he says that if she must
use birth control, he will put her on the pill. "No," she
insists. She doesn't trust the high estrogen levels—
she's read the research, newly unearthed by women
health activists, about the heightened risk of strokes,
heart attacks, blood clots. "Oh, that's just a bunch of
feminist hysteria," he says. "No it isn't," she says, crossing her arms. "I want a diaphragm." She gets it. Some
years later, the data compiled by "feminist hysterics"

proves to be scientific and overwhelming. The pill's manufacturers, convinced of the dangers, reduce the estrogen dose by a third.

The young woman, of course, is me, and this story serves as full disclosure. I can't write a preface to one of the early and essential texts of the '70s women's health movement without admitting the bias of my personal gratitude. And I can't read Barbara Ehrenreich and Deirdre English's *Complaints and Disorders* without being consumed all over again with excitement about the era these pages recall: a time when feminists challenged a male medical establishment that had for so long withheld information and told women how to think and feel about their bodies; a time when women collectively reframed the questions, re-examined the history, reassessed the data, and reinforced each other's efforts to change the system; a time when a critical mass of women came to understand that seeing and thinking for themselves was fundamental to their liberation. As Deirdre English says of the book she and Ehrenreich self-published and shipped out in Barbara's children's old Pampers boxes in the early '70s, "The most important moral point is: women defining their own needs, not having their needs 'constructed' by the political interests of anyone else—men, doctors, psychiatrists, the state, the Tea Party, anything but women themselves."

Complaints and Disorders is a profound act of independent and historical investigation. Its two authors were posing questions no one had asked, inspecting archives no one had read, and charting a terrain no one had mapped. The revelations their work yielded remain central to feminist analysis and contemporary women's self-understanding. Ehrenreich and English were drilling down through cultural sedimentary layers to bedrock. They wanted to know how we got from there to here: What is the nature of the relationship between women and their doctors and why is it that way? How has the medical world come to define femininity in a particular fashion? How did doctors become the über-guardians of sexist ideology?

"In writing this, we have tried to see beyond our own experiences (and anger)," they wrote, "and to understand medical sexism as a *social force* helping to shape the options and social roles of all women." That is, they looked to the connective tissue between individual women and social institutions and between our present condition and our Victorian past. And what they uncovered was a long hidden history shaped by complex social, political, and economic dynamics.

They found the crucial prequel to the troubling tale of modern women and modern medicine.

With the ascendancy of a male medical establishment in the second half of the nineteenth century, physicians took over the role of the clergy, regulating women's reproduction and thereby defining women as the compromised, defective sex. While the church fathers justified their control over women with the contention that the weaker sex "naturally" lacked morals, the medical men rested their case on women's "natural" lack of health. *Medicine's prime contribution to sexist ideology,* Ehrenreich and English emphasized, *"has been to describe women as sick, and as potentially sickening to men."* The new "scientific" terms were in no way an improvement over the old moral basis for control. Quite the contrary. "The fading of the last vestiges of religious moralism from scientific ideology has made it all the more mystifying, all the more effective as a potential tool for domination."

Ehrenreich and English saw their work as a starting point—they were looking to open a much larger inquiry, conducted by other women who were, likewise, framing their own questions, thinking for themselves. "We trust that you take what we have done not as a final statement but as an invitation to go much further," they wrote, addressing their readers directly with a refreshing openness. And in the years to follow, many feminist investigators and researchers took up the call, limning the untold story of women's health. Scholars of women's history—particularly those who came out of the school of social history pursued from the ground up—would push deeper into the thickets of Victorian women's experience and return with the trophies of original research and catalyzing insight. Carroll Smith-Rosenberg's *Disorderly Conduct*, which explored Victorian women's efforts to resist the medical and cultural straitjackets of their times, and Elaine Showalter's *The Female Malady*, a feminist examination of the history of psychiatry from Victorian to modern times, are just two notable examples of many such works that emerged in the course of the '70s and '80s. (As is Ehrenreich and English's *For Her Own Good*, their wonderfully witty and classic chronicle of the two-hundred-year history of medical, psychiatric, and parenting "advice" literature directed at American women.)

But my other emotion in rereading *Complaints and Disorders* is melancholy. Because it is this very kind of work—historical, real-world, accessible, driven by a concern for women's conditions and a desire to change them, seeking to inspire other feminist researchers—that has suffered in the shift to a more abstract and abstruse approach to gender studies. Ehrenreich and English were widening the lens to investigate an entire social system—its history, its mechanisms, its consequences. More and more, though, gender studies, constrained by the demands of academic life and the vogues of a postmodern age, has narrowed the aperture, making increasingly pinched arguments stripped of material reality, and sometimes comprehensible only to the scholastic circle that knows the rarified code.

Ehrenreich and English wrote to be understood by the largest world of women possible—they were not appealing to a tenure committee. Their prose is full of urgency, passion, and, at the same time, utter respect for the complicated and contradictory historical channels they were navigating. It was important to them to be as clear and honest and true to their findings as possible, because they knew it was important to the lives of real women, to the society they lived in and its prospects for change. They were committed both to social justice and historical integrity, and intent on compromising neither.

Contemporary scholars have taken second-wave feminists to task for universalizing women's situation. In particular, the criticism "You didn't look at race and class" has become a familiar *j'accuse* leveled against an older generation of feminist theorists and writers. And it is a deserved corrective in many cases. But when I returned to Ehrenreich and English's book after some years, what I found most striking was their determination to do just that—not as an addendum or a "to be sure" caveat, but as the fundament of their analysis. The very first sentence of their first chapter reads: "Women are not a 'class'; they are not uniformly oppressed; they do not all experience sexism in the same ways." In fact, the rapidly polarizing economic scene of late industrializing nineteenth-century America, they noted, divided women by race and class as never before—and defined them, medically, in diametrically opposed terms.

From beginning to end, *Complaints and Disorders* is a systematic exploration of race and class dynamics and how they shaped the conditions and relations of American women: how these divisions were defined by the economy, manipulated by the culture, exploited by medical practitioners, and, maybe most disturbing, enforced by women themselves. You can't begin to understand the medical sexism of the late eighteen hundreds, Ehrenreich and English argued, until you understand the way these divisions were represented—and, crucially, misrepresented—by the rising medical patriarchs.

"For the affluent women, society prescribed lives of leisured indolence; for the working-class women, backbreaking toil. No *single* ideology of sexism could embrace both realities or justify both social roles." The realities, which *Complaints and Disorders* limns with vivid examples (and striking illustrations from the time), were far higher rates of maternal mortality, failing health, and contagious illness among working-class immigrant and black women than their affluent sisters, thanks to working women's punishing hours of labor, grim living conditions, and poor nutrition. These were realities the Victorian physicians chose to ignore for their own purposes; in fact, they flipped them on their heads to pathologize women of the class they wished to treat. The doctors "reversed the causality and found the soft, 'civilized' life of the upper classes more health-threatening and medically interesting than hard work and privation." The ailments they found most "interesting" involved affluent women's sex organs. According to the new medical men, the cure for all that ailed the upper-class white angel of the house, particularly the mental ills of neurasthenia and hysteria brought on by her restricted hothouse life, could be located in her private parts. Treatment invariably required uterine invasion, from leeches applied to the cervix to ovariotomies (or "female castration"), thousands of which were performed in the late nineteenth century. Defining bourgeois women as the sickest of their sex also served physicians' economic interests: by claiming these supposedly desperately ill women needed special care that only "highly trained" (male) physicians could provide, they both undercut their main competition—self-taught female midwives and healers—and cultivated a female clientele whose wealthy husbands could foot the bill.

Meanwhile, the doctors declared the immigrant and black woman of the lower classes to be healthy as a (work) horse, naturally fit for superhuman levels of sweat and travail. A popular medical authority at the time, Dr. Lucien Warner (just one of the many choice "experts" Ehrenreich and English uncovered in their research) wrote in 1874, "The African negress, who toils beside her husband in the fields of the south, and Bridget, who washes and scrubs and toils in our homes at the north, enjoy for the most part good health, with comparative immunity from uterine disease." The new male practitioners may not have found these women too sick to work, Ehrenreich and English observed, but they *did* find them to be the prime bearers of bad health, human vectors of disease and dirt who needed to be monitored, controlled, and quarantined. They were joined in that view by their self-appointed publicists in the new mass media, who rushed to sound the alarms. Garments sewn by tenement sweatshop women were teeming with germs! Domestic servants were carrying deadly afflictions into the bowers of domestic gentility! Mary Mallon, the Irish American cook more infamously known as "Typhoid Mary," became the most wanted poster girl of pestilence criminality, an exemplar of "biological guerrilla warfare at its most virulent," Ehrenreich and English wryly remarked. That virulence was happily amplified by the penny press, which cast Mallon as "a fiend popping human skulls into a skillet."

One of the many great insights of this book is the authors' recognition that the distinction the Victorian doctors enforced between rich and poor women mirrored a much older duality in cultural demonizations of women. "Beneath all this," they wrote, "ran two ancient strands of sexist ideology: contempt for women as weak and defective, and fear of women as dangerous and polluting. Here we see the two separated, and applied to wealthy and poor females respectively. Upper- and upper-middle-class women were 'sick'; working-class women were 'sickening.'" By assigning these two reigning canards to two different classes of women, the physicians had dodged the contradictions. And assured a divide-and-conquer outcome.

These divisions were damaging to both classes of women—and ultimately to the movement that might have liberated them from the thrall of medical misogyny. As Ehrenreich and English so painfully showed, women's health reformers of the turn of the century failed to challenge that divide in any meaningful way. Worse, they relied on it to justify their cause. They were breaking out of their housebound, helpless-female status—so as to better control and quarantine their polluted sisters.

Contemporary critics like to claim that feminist chroniclers have "covered up" this ugly chapter, concealed the racism and classism that dogged the end of the first wave of the women's movement. But here again, the denouncers would do well to reread *Complaints and Disorders*. Ehrenreich and English did not flinch from examining the part that race- and class-based eugenic arguments played in disfiguring the birth-control campaigns of the early 1900s. They traced the devolution of a bourgeois women's health reform effort that "began to make frank appeal to upper-middle-class self-interest" and that accused poor and non-white women of every woe from poverty to feeble-mindedness. They quoted representatives of the American Birth Control League and other privileged enclaves of women's health advocacy whose arguments were "explicitly racist." And they concluded that feminist health activists—no matter how successful their individual efforts to free themselves from the Victorian cult of female frailty—sold their movement down the river by refusing to interrogate their own flattering Lady Bountiful self-image:

> The upper-middle-class woman activist of the 1890s and early twentieth century had left her sisters far behind on their chaise longues, in sick rooms and health spas. She had rejected a medical ideology that defined her as sick and confined her to uselessness. But she seems to have won "release" only on condition that she both remain true to the interests of her class and take on social roles that were extensions of the wife/mother role, as social worker or volunteer "uplifter." . . .
>
> The issue of health—female health and family health—which potentially could have united women of different classes, now divided them into reformers on one side and "problems" on the other.

WHAT HAD CHANGED BY THE TIME EHRENREICH and English first published their book? "Very little," they concluded. The days of leeches and ovariotomies were long gone, but the relationship between women and the medical system was still locked in many of the same destructive dynamics, with pregnancy still treated like a medical affliction, hysterectomies performed at the drop of a hat (as much as 50 percent of them unnecessarily), and women's dependence on doctors—and the medical industry's withholding of information—greater than ever before. "In the '70s," Ehrenreich reminded me recently, "you couldn't get information even on the hormonal cycle. Information that would seem like sixth grade sex ed material was unavailable—and practically illicit." Even feminist gains were being pounced on by the medical profession as new opportunities for control. "Doctors moved in on each sexual or reproductive right as soon as it was liberated," Ehrenreich and English noted. "They now control abortion and almost all reliable means of contraception. Even sexual unresponsiveness—the 'natural' condition of our great-grandmothers—has become a medical problem, with its own sex 'clinics' and its own brand of medical specialists."

Most significant, the relationship between women and the medical system was still ruled by an unchallenged race and class divide. "Middle- and upper-class women are still a 'client caste' to the medical profession," they wrote, while lower-income women can't get the most basic health care.

> The fragmented pattern of public health services for low-income women—here a VD clinic, there a Planned Parenthood clinic, almost nowhere a low-cost comprehensive care center—shows that they are still treated more as public health problems than as human beings needing individualized medical care. For no groups is this truer than for black, Puerto Rican, and Chicana women. Once lumped together with Italians, Poles, and other immigrant groups as "inferior stock," Third World women now stand almost alone as the special target of such population control measures as involuntary sterilization.

But as Ehrenreich and English were finishing *Complaints and Disorders* in the early '70s, they were hopeful that a new crop of politicized women might, at long last, challenge the class barrier in medicine. "There is very little danger today that middle-class women will relate to poor and working-class women purely as missionaries or 'organizers' for health reforms because middle-class women are becoming so acutely aware of their *own* oppression in the medical system," they wrote. "The growth of feminist consciousness gives us the possibility, for the first time, of a truly egalitarian, mass women's health movement."

Complaints and Disorders was published in 1973, the same year as the Supreme Court's decision on *Roe v. Wade*, legalizing abortion. By 1976, Congress had passed the Hyde Amendment, which banned Medicaid funding for abortions for low-income women. Which is to say, within three short years, abortion went from a basic health right for all women to a class privilege. And remained that way. As I write this thirty-five years later, Republican Congressman Joe Pitts, who co-authored the Stupak Amendment (denying federal money to insurance plans covering abortion), has just been named chairman of the key House health panel that has jurisdiction over women's medical care and Medicaid. The new Speaker of the House, Rep. John A. Boehner, an adamant opponent of legal abortion, has just paid tribute to "one of my all-time heroes": Rep. Henry J. Hyde, the architect of the Hyde Amendment. And Republicans in Congress want to defund Planned Parenthood, an essential provider of family planning services for low-income women, and deny aid to millions of low-income women for prenatal care, contraception, breast and cervical cancer screenings, HIV testing, and nutritional support for their newborns.

A women's health movement committed to crossing class and race lines did, to some extent, emerge in the '70s. You could see it in the early struggles by feminist activists to create community-based clinics in low-income neighborhoods, to fight coerced sterilizations of poor and minority women, and to protest the use of experimental birth control drugs on women in impoverished countries and the dumping of pharmaceuticals damaging to women's fertility in Third World nations. But these efforts were scattered and fragile, pursued in fits and starts and vulnerable to longstanding divisions and resentments. By the '80s and '90s, as women's health advocates became consumed with fighting rear-guard actions against the rising force of the anti-abortion New Right, as a laywomen's movement became "professionalized" and subsumed by well-heeled nonprofit organizations, as access to health insurance became increasingly a class privilege, and, maybe most pernicious, as women's health concerns were increasingly defined in narrowly individualistic terms, these fragile bridges built across the race and class divide began to crumble. When a grassroots international women's health movement emerged in the '80s, largely in reaction to the discriminatory and patronizing policies practiced by the United States and other Western countries in developing nations, its visionaries, leaders, and foot soldiers came mostly from the so-called Third World; the role of American women health activists was marginal and, at best, supplemental.

Ehrenreich and English marveled at "the endless plasticity of a medical 'science' that can adjust its theories for age, sex, or social class, depending on the needs of time." In our present moment, that plasticity is on ample display in the invention of new complaints and disorders, new lifestyle maladies for an image-obsessed age that the medical industry—and its powerful sidekick Big Pharma – can respond to and exploit. Yet again, these are ailments conceived only with an upper-class female demographic in mind, as are their luxury "cures": hormone replacement therapy, cosmetic surgery, Lap-Band operations, collagen implants, Botox injections, vaginal reconstruction, and Viagra-esque medications for "female sexual dysfunction," to name just a few. Yet again, medical publicists co-opt feminist rhetoric to market their wares. Their procedures and regimens, they promise, serve the needs of "the liberated woman," elevating her "self-esteem," enhancing her "freedom of choice," arming her with the tools of "self-empowerment." "It's your body," plastic surgery ads advise. "Shouldn't you be in charge of how it looks?"

Contemporary pharmaceutical and medical appeals to women merge seamlessly with the offerings of a media awash in women's "well-being" programs, reality makeover shows, and health magazines promising a transformational path to female "independence" that invariably routes its consumers through a Monopoly board of drugstore, doctor's office, and surgery ward. The Victorian medical industry's habit of aggravating upper-class women's health anxieties by concocting ever more dubious diseases for them to fear is hardly behind us, as the many all-points bulletins in the "women's health" media on repressed libido syndromes, kitchen counter killer germs, and arcane food intolerances attest. "Low sexual desire?" *Health* magazine asks its female readers. They better consult a "sexual medicine specialist"—it could be nerve damage, a broken thyroid, high blood pressure, diabetes. "What's lurking in your DNA?" *Women's Health* magazine frets—in the same line-up that offers "The Enemy Inside You: Chronic inflammation—a slow, silent disturbance that never shuts off," and "Dangerous Personal Trainers—they are putting your life at risk."

In the meantime, low-income women still lack

access to the most basic health and reproductive care. And this at a time when 16.4 million women are living in poverty, the highest number since the census began keeping count in 1966. Female poverty rates are rapidly rising, and rising fastest among women of color. Even before the recession hit, low-income women were four times more likely than their higher-income sisters to report fair to poor health. Nearly 40 percent of Latina women and a quarter of black women lack health insurance. One-third of Latina and black women report being forced to delay or forego health care for financial reasons in the preceding year (compared with one-fourth of their white counterparts). And one-fourth of all women can't fill a necessary medical prescription because they can't afford it. In 2010, the latest study by the federal Department of Health and Human Services' "Healthy People Agenda" found that *most* of the benchmarks of women's basic health had not been met.

At least the modern crop of female health activists aren't handmaidens to the medical industry like their Victorian antecedents. Or so it seems. They have, after all, challenged medical sexism in many important respects. Drug trials and longitudinal health studies are no longer conducted only on men. Class-action suits supported by feminist efforts have banished harmful pregnancy drugs and contraceptives from DES to the Dalkon Shield IUD. Women's health research now receives federal funding. The National Institutes of Health has an initiative on women's health. Surgeons can't make the unilateral decision to do a radical mastectomy while the patient is still under the anesthesia. Medical professors no longer routinely include *Playboy* centerfolds in their anatomy slides. Half of medical school students are now women, and the proportion of female physicians has risen from less than 8 percent in 1970 to almost 30 percent today. None of these milestones were arrived at without a fierce and sustained battle on the part of feminist activists.

But have female health crusaders truly declared their independence from the medical system, or are they still, in ways we have failed to come to terms with, unwittingly complicit? Few are making a clear-eyed assessment of this treacherous present moment. Barbara Ehrenreich is one of the rare exceptions. In her 2001 *Harper's* essay, "Welcome to Cancerland," later revisited in her 2009 book, *Bright-Sided: How the Relentless Promotion of Positive Thinking Has Undermined America*, she pondered the eclipse of a grassroots campaign for breast cancer research by "huge, corporate-sponsored, pink gatherings" where post-op women are invited to "Shop for the Cure," run 10Ks in

T-shirts emblazoned with corporate and pharmaceutical logos, accessorize with "angel pins," and cuddle with "Wish Upon a Star Bears." What was once independent activism has morphed into "a ladies' auxiliary to the cancer-industrial complex," Ehrenreich wrote.

> And although we may imagine ourselves to be well past the era of patriarchal medicine, obedience is the message behind the infantilizing theme in breast-cancer culture, as represented by the teddy bears, the crayons, and the prevailing pinkness. You are encouraged to regress to a little-girl state, to suspend critical judgment, and to accept whatever measures the doctors, as parent surrogates, choose to impose.

Ehrenreich wrote these words out of political and personal experience, both hard-won—as a lifelong health activist and as someone who had, just a year earlier, undergone treatment for breast cancer.

Lurking behind the infantilization she describes is a political imperative, one that is not comforting to modern feminism for all the progress we've made. So much of our current "raised consciousness" seems to focus on body issues, but not as Ehrenreich and English focused on them. The gap between concern for bodies and concern for the body politic has, in some ways, never been wider. It's as if *Our Bodies Ourselves*, that formative and transformative document of the '70s women's health movement, has degenerated into *I Am My Body*. We concentrate on appearance, our "right" to display, and our urge to prettify at the expense of economic and political analyses, as Ehrenreich and English warned in the closing pages of *Complaints and Disorders:*

> There is no way for us to come to terms with our own bodies. . .because, when you come right down to it, our *bodies* are not the issue. Biology is not the issue. The issue is power, in all the ways it affects us. . . .To act on this understanding is to ask for more than "control over our own bodies." It is to ask for, and struggle for, control over the social options available to us, and control over all the institutions of society that now define those options.

We might want to believe that after nearly forty years, *Complaints and Disorders* is outdated, but we do so at our peril.

February 2011

Complaints
and
Disorders

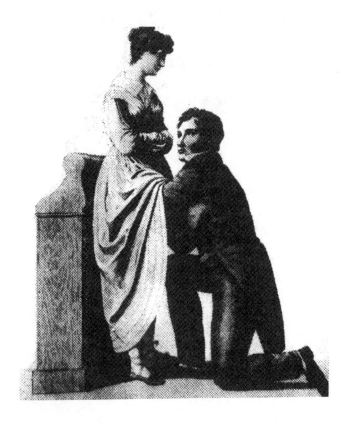

Gynecological exam

Introduction: A Perspective on the Social Role of Medicine

THE MEDICAL SYSTEM IS STRATEGIC FOR WOMEN'S liberation. It is the guardian of reproductive technology—birth control, abortion, and the means for safe childbirth. It holds the promise of freedom from hundreds of unspoken fears and complaints that have handicapped women throughout history. When we demand control over our own bodies, we are making that demand above all to the medical system. It is the keeper of the keys.

But the medical system is also strategic to women's oppression. Medical science has been one of the most powerful sources of sexist ideology in our culture. Justifications for sexual discrimination—in education, in jobs, in public life—must ultimately rest on the one thing that differentiates women from men: their bodies. Theories of male superiority ultimately rest on biology.

Medicine stands between biology and social policy, between the "mysterious" world of the laboratory and everyday life. It makes public interpretations of biological theory; it dispenses the medical fruits of scientific advances. Biology discovers hormones; doctors make public judgments on whether "hormonal imbalances" make women unfit for public office. More generally, biology traces the origins of disease; doctors pass judgment on who is sick and who is well.

Medicine's prime contribution to sexist ideology has been to describe women as sick, and as potentially sickening to men.

Of course, medicine did not invent sexism. The view that women are "sick," or defective versions of men, is as old as Eden. In the traditions of Western thought, man represents wholeness, strength, and health. Woman is a "misbegotten male," weak and incomplete. Since Hippocrates bewailed women's "perpetual infirmities," medicine has only echoed the prevailing male sentiment: it has treated pregnancy and menopause as diseases, menstruation as a chronic disorder, childbirth as a surgical event. At the same time, woman's "weakness" has never barred her from heavy labor;

her "instability" has never disqualified her from total responsibility for child raising.

In the psychology of sexism, contempt is always mixed with *fear*. If woman is sick, there is always the danger that she will infect men. Menstrual and post-partum taboos, which serve to protect males from female "impurity," are almost universal in human cultures and, not surprisingly, are strictest in the most patriarchal societies. Historically, medicine ratified the dangers of women by describing women as the source of venereal disease. Today, we are more likely to be viewed as mental health hazards—emasculating men and destructively dominating children.

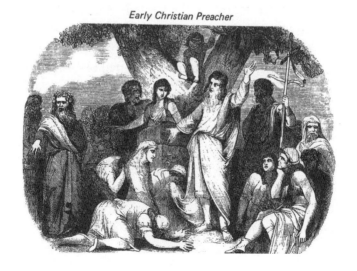

Early Christian Preacher

Medicine inherited from religion its role as a guardian of sexist ideology. Early Christian writings are filled with denunciations of women as men's spiritual inferiors, their contagious sexuality capable of dragging men down into the mire of passion. "Every woman ought to be filled with shame at the thought that she is a woman," wrote Clement of Alexandria (c. 150–215). And St. John Chrysostom (c. 347–407)—an early church father who once pushed a woman off a cliff to demonstrate his immunity to temptation—said, "Among all the savage beasts none is found so harmful as woman." In medieval Europe, it was the Church that regulated women's reproductivity, legislating on abortion and contraception, proscribing the use of herbs to ease the pain of labor. It banned women from the sacraments during menstruation and the weeks following delivery. It controlled the licensing of midwives and, in some cases, that of physicians generally.

American Protestantism also resisted the legalization of contraception and abortion and even the use of anesthesia in labor. But generally it took a more benign and paternalistic view of women. It granted them spirituality though only at the price of their sexuality. It granted them "equality" if they stayed within their "God-appointed sphere" of domestic life. And Protestantism, unlike Catholicism, was willing to join forces with science in discovering and upholding the "natural order" of things. Nineteenth-century religious leaders happily supplemented religious justifications of sexism with newly developed biomedical ones. Gradually woman's supposed physical infirmities won out over her moral defects as the rationale for male supremacy. The secularization of male domination has advanced rapidly in just the last few decades: contraception is legal *when dispensed by doctors.* Abortion is no longer a moral outrage but a matter "between a woman *and her doctor.*"

Thus it is no accident that the women's liberation movement today puts so much emphasis on health and "body" issues. Women are dependent on the medical system for the most basic control over their own reproductivity. At the same time, women's encounters with the medical system bring them face to face with sexism in its most unmistakably crude and insulting forms.

Our motivation to write this pamphlet comes out of our own experiences as women, as health care consumers, and as activists in the women's health movement. In writing this, we have tried to see beyond our own experiences (and anger) and to understand medi-

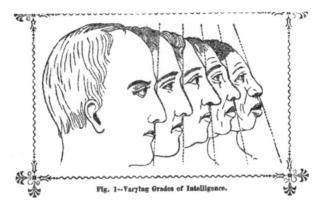

Fig. 1--Varying Grades of Intelligence.

1891 scientific illustration of ethnic differences

cal sexism as a *social force* helping to shape the options and social roles of all women.

Our approach is largely historical. In the first sections of this pamphlet we attempt to describe medicine's contribution to sexist ideology and sexual oppression in the late nineteenth and early twentieth centuries (approximately 1865 to 1920 though a few of the important medical books were written earlier). We chose to begin with this period because it witnessed a pronounced shift from a religious to a biomedical rationale for sexism, as well as the formation of the medical profession as we know it—a male elite with a legal monopoly over medical practice. We feel that this period provides a perspective essential for understanding our relation to the modern medical system. In the last two sections we attempt to apply that perspective to our present situation and the issues that concern us today.

We want to make it clear that we have not tried to write a definite social history of women and medicine in America, nor have we tried to make an objective evaluation of women's health or the quality of their medical treatment, past or present. Our interest is primarily in medical *ideas* about women, particularly the ideas and themes that struck a chord with *us* and seemed to explain our own condition. We trust that you will take what we have done not as a final statement but as an invitation to go much further.

In this pamphlet our focus is on women and their relation to medical practice and medical beliefs. But the context goes beyond medicine itself and embraces all oppressed groups. In the historical period we have studied, science in general was invoked to justify the social inequities imposed by race and class as well as by sex. Industrial technology—plus the labor of millions of working people—was creating the wealth of the business elite that still rules America. If technology could make some men rich and powerful, surely *science* could justify their power. Racism, like sexism, seemed to shift from the realm of prejudice into the light of "objective" science. Blacks and European immigrants were described as congenitally inferior to white Anglo-Saxon Protestants, having smaller brains, larger muscles, and a host of "inherited" social traits. Race and class oppression, like sexual oppression, were not undemocratic; they were only "natural."

During this transitional period morality was still mixed with science in the ideology of domination. Scientists believed that moral traits—like the supposed shiftlessness of blacks or disorderliness of Irish immigrants—were inheritable. Public health officials spoke of "God's sanitary laws," and doctors saw themselves as the moral, as well as physical, guardians of women. Today the transition is almost complete: science needs no assistance from the pulpit. When it passes judgment on the IQ of blacks, or on the prenatally determined psychological differences between the sexes, it is only being "objective." The fading of the last vestiges of religious moralism from scientific ideology has made it all the more mystifying, all the more effective as a potential tool for domination. We hope that the story presented here will contribute to people's confidence and ability to see through the "rational," "scientific" disguises of power.

Women and Medicine in the Late Nineteenth and Early Twentieth Centuries

THE HISTORICAL SETTING

Women are not a "class"; they are not uniformly oppressed; they do not all experience sexism in the same ways. In the period between 1865 and 1920, class differences among American women were particularly sharp: the lifestyle, manners, and expectations of upper-class women had little in common with those of working-class women. This was a period of rapid industrialization, urbanization, and class polarization, affecting all Americans. In the cities—and here we are concerned only with the urban world, where medical trends were set—two classes, essentially new to American society, were coming to dominate the scene:

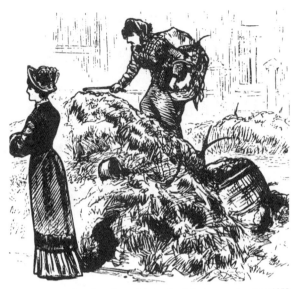

Female garbage-picker and well-to-do passerby, about 1875

an upper middle class whose wealth was based on business and industry and an industrial working class whose labor provided that wealth.*

The social roles of women in these two classes were almost diametrically opposed. For the affluent women, society prescribed lives of leisured indolence;

*It is important not to project current conceptions of class onto the classes of the late nineteenth and early twentieth centuries. The urban working class of the time bore no relation to today's Archie Bunker image of the working class (which is inaccurate today anyway). Mostly European immigrants, they were extremely poor, even by the standards of the day. They occupied somewhat the same social status as poor urban blacks do today.

for the working-class women, backbreaking toil. No *single* ideology of sexism could embrace both realities or justify both social roles. Hence, biomedical thought had to provide two distinct views of women: one appropriate to the upper middle class (and the middle class that aspired to an upper-middle-class lifestyle), and one appropriate to poor and working-class women.

It was as if there were two different human species of females. Affluent women were seen as inherently sick, too weak and delicate for anything but the mildest pastimes, while working-class women were believed to be inherently healthy and robust. The reality was very different. Working-class women, who put in long hours of work and received inadequate rest and nutrition, suffered far more than wealthy women from contagious diseases and complications of childbirth.

But doctors reversed the causality and found the soft, "civilized" life of the upper classes more health-threatening and medically interesting than hard work and privation. Dr. Lucien Warner, a popular medical authority,* wrote in 1874, "It is not then hard work and privation which make the women of our coun-

---

*We have chosen to quote only those doctors who seemed to us to be representative, based on our reading of popular gynecology books in the collection of the New York Academy of Medicine.

try invalids, but circumstances and habits intimately connected with the so-called blessings of wealth and refinement." In an article on the servant shortage, a contemporary journalist in *The Nation* (1912) wrote:

> It might be a very good thing for a woman's health to sweep her room, and make her bed, and dust her parlor, and get her dinner; but the attenuation of her physical energies has been carried so far by civilization that it will take a generation or two of golfing, boating and bathing to give her sex back the strength of old days, when the domestic virtues went hand in hand with the domestic labors.

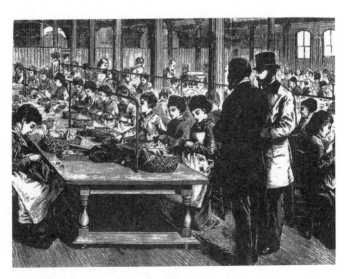

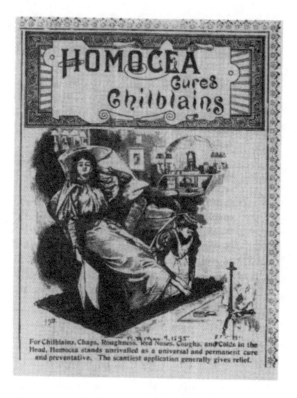

For Chilblains, Chaps, Roughness, Red Noses, Coughs, and Colds in the Head, Homocea stands unrivalled as a universal and permanent cure and preventative. The scantiest application generally gives relief.

Someone had to be well enough to do the work, though, and working-class women, Dr. Warner noted with relief, were *not* invalids: "The African negress, who toils beside her husband in the fields of the south, and Bridget, who washes, and scrubs and toils in our homes at the north, enjoy for the most part good health, with comparative immunity from uterine disease."

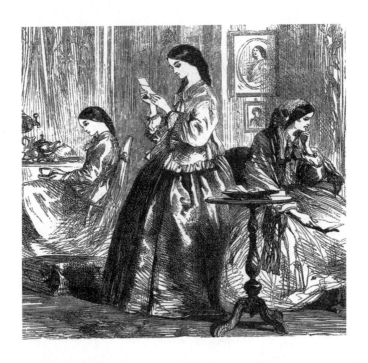

But if "Bridget" and "Beulah" were not too sick to do the housework and the factory work, they *were* unhealthy—at least to the upper-class observers who described immigrants and blacks as congenitally dirty and possibly contagious. The working-class woman might not faint, or get "uterine disease," but she undoubtedly harbored germs of typhoid, cholera, or venereal disease. Furthermore, as a breeder, she was seen as a public health threat, undermining the American "race" with her "inferior" offspring.

Beneath all this ran two ancient strands of sexist ideology: contempt for women as weak and defective, and fear of women as dangerous and polluting. Here we see the two separated, and applied to wealthy and poor females respectively. Upper- and upper-middle-class women were "sick"; working-class women were "sickening." In the sections that follow we deal first with the upper-middle-class or "sick" women, their relation to the medical system and the ideology applied to them, and then we go on to the biomedical views of the working class, and working-class women in particular.

The "Sick" Women
of the Upper Classes

THE AFFLUENT WOMAN NORMALLY SPENT A HUSHED
and peaceful life indoors, sewing, sketching and reading romances, planning menus and supervising servants and children. Her clothes, a sort of portable
prison of tight corsets and long skirts, prevented
activity any more vigorous than a Sunday stroll. Society agreed that she was frail and sickly. Her delicate
nervous system had to be shielded as carefully as her
body, for the slightest shock could send her reeling
off to bed. Elizabeth Barrett Browning, for example, although she was an extraordinarily productive
woman, spent six years in bed following her brother's
death in a sailboat accident.

But not even the most sheltered woman lived in a
vacuum. Just outside the suffocating world of the par-

lor and the boudoir lay a world of industrial horror. This was the period of America's industrial revolution, a revolution based on the ruthless exploitation of working people. Women, and children as young as six, worked fourteen-hour days in factories and sweatshops for sub-subsistence wages. Labor struggles were violent—bordering, at times, on civil wars. For businessmen, too, survival was a bitter struggle: you squeezed what you could out of the workers, screwed the competition, and the devil take the hindmost. Fortunes were

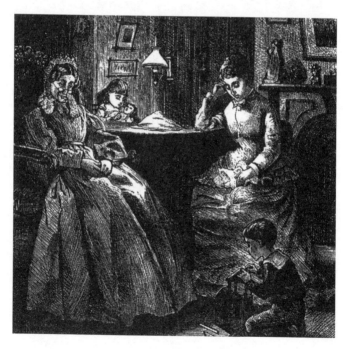

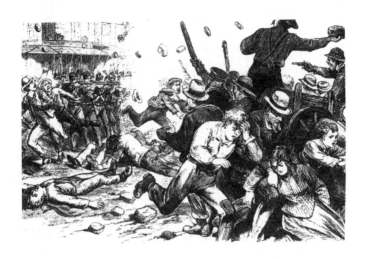

made and destroyed overnight, and with them rode the fates of thousands of smaller businessmen.

The genteel lady of leisure was not just an anomaly in an otherwise dog-eat-dog world. She was as much a product of that world as her husband or his employees. It was the wealth extracted in that harsh outside world that enabled a man to afford a totally leisured wife. She was the social ornament that proved a man's success: her idleness, her delicacy, her childlike ignorance of "reality" gave a man the "class" that money alone could not provide. And it was the very harshness of the outside world that led men to see the home as a refuge—"a sacred place, a vestal temple," a "tent pitch'd in a world not right," presided over by a gentle, ethereal wife. Among the affluent classes, the worlds of men and women drifted further and further apart, with divergent standards of decorum, of health, of morality itself.

There were exceptional women in the upper classes—women who rebelled against the life of enforced leisure, the limitations on meaningful work—and it is these exceptional women who usually are remembered in history books. Many became women's rights activists or social reformers. A brave few struggled to make their way in the professions. And toward the end of the nineteenth century a growing number were demanding, and getting, college educations. But the majority of upper- and upper-middle-class women had little chance to make independent lives for themselves; they were financially at the mercy of husbands or fathers. They had to accept their roles—outwardly at least—and remain dutifully housebound, white-gloved and ornamental. Of course, only a small minority of urban women could afford a life of total leisure, but a great many more women in the middle class aspired to it and did their best to live like "ladies."

THE CULT OF FEMALE INVALIDISM

The boredom and confinement of affluent women fostered a morbid cult of hypochondria—"female invalidism"—that began in the mid-nineteenth century and did not completely fade until the late 1910s. Sickness pervaded upper- and upper-middle-class female culture. Health spas and female specialists sprung up everywhere and became part of the regular circuit of fashionable women. And in the 1850s a steady stream of popular home readers by doctors appeared, all

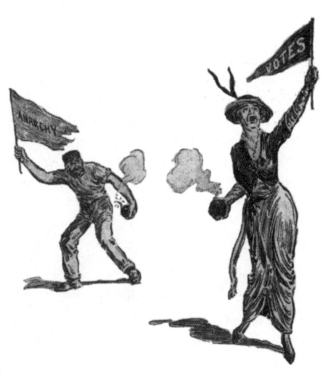

on the subject of female health. Literature aimed at female readers lingered on the romantic pathos of illness and death; popular women's magazines featured such stories as "The Grave of My Friend" and "Song of Dying." Paleness and lassitude (along with filmy white gowns) came into vogue. It was acceptable, even fashionable, to retire to bed with "sick headaches," "nerves," and a host of other mysterious ailments.

In response, feminist writers and female doctors expressed their dismay at the chronic invalidism of affluent women. Dr. Mary Putnam Jacobi, an outstanding woman doctor of the late nineteenth century, wrote in 1895:

> . . . it is considered natural and almost laudable to break down under all conceivable varieties of strain—a winter dissipation, a houseful of servants, a quarrel with a female friend, not to speak of more legitimate reasons. . . . Women who expect to go to bed every menstrual period expect to collapse if by chance they find themselves on their feet for a few hours during such a crisis. Constantly considering their nerves, urged to consider them by well-intentioned but shortsighted advisors, they pretty soon become nothing but a bundle of nerves.

Charlotte Perkins Gilman, the feminist writer and economist, concluded bitterly that American men "have bred a race of women weak enough to be handed about like invalids; or mentally weak enough to pretend they are—and to like it."

It is impossible to tell, in retrospect, how sick upper-middle-class women really were. Life expectancies for women were slightly higher than for men though the difference was nowhere near as great as it is today.

It is true, however, that women—*all* women—faced certain risks that men did not share, or share to the same degree. First were the risks associated with childbearing, which were all the greater in an age of primitive obstetrical technique when little was known about the importance of prenatal nutrition. In 1915 (the first year for which national figures are available) 61 women died for every 10,000 live babies born, compared to 2 per 10,000 today, and the maternal mortality rates were doubtless higher in the nineteenth century. Without adequate, and usually without any, means of contraception, a married woman could expect to face the risk of childbirth repeatedly through her fertile years. After each childbirth a women might suffer any number of gynecological complications, such as a prolapsed (slipped) uterus or irreparable pelvic tear, which would stay with her for the rest of her life.

Another special risk to women came with tuberculosis, the "white plague." In the mid-nineteenth century, TB raged at epidemic proportions, and it continued to be a major threat until well into the twentieth century. Everyone was affected, but women, especially young women, were particularly vulnerable, often dying at rates twice as high as those of men of their age group. For every hundred women aged twenty in 1865, more than five would be dead from TB by the age of thirty, and more than eight would be dead by the age of fifty.

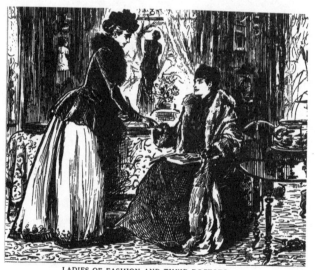

LADIES OF FASHION AND THEIR DOCTORS
(Scene: The Waiting-Room of a Fashionable Physician.)

Fair Patient (*just ushered in*).—" What—*you* here, Lizzie ? Why, ain't you *well?*"
Second Ditto.—" Perfectly, tnanks! But what's the matter with *you*, dear?"
First Ditto.—" Oh, nothing whatever! I'm as right as possible, dearest . . .!"

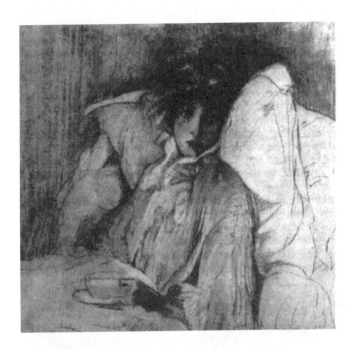

(It is now believed that hormonal changes associated with puberty and childbearing accounted for the greater vulnerability of young women to TB.)

The dangers of childbearing, and of TB, must have shadowed women's lives in a way we no longer know. But these dangers cannot explain the cultural phenomenon of "female invalidism" which, unlike TB and maternal mortality, was confined to women of a particular social class. The most important legitimization of this fashion came not from the actual dangers faced by women but from the medical profession.

The medical view of women's health not only acknowledged the specific risks associated with reproductivity, it went much further: it identified *all* female functions as *inherently* sick. Puberty was seen as a "crisis," throwing the entire female organism into turmoil. Menstruation—or the lack of it—was regarded as pathological throughout a woman's life. Dr. W. C. Taylor, in his book *A Physician's Counsels to Woman in Health and Disease* (1871), gave a warning typical of those found in popular health books of the time:

> We cannot too emphatically urge the importance of regarding these monthly returns as periods of ill health, as days when the ordinary occupations are to be suspended or modified . . . Long walks, dancing, shopping, riding and parties should be avoided at this time of the month invariably and under all circumstances. . . . Another reason why every woman should look upon herself as an invalid once a month, is that the monthly flow aggravates any existing affection of the womb and readily rekindles the expiring flames of disease.

Similarly, a pregnant woman was "indisposed," and doctors campaigned against the practice of midwifery on the grounds that pregnancy was a disease and demanded the care of a doctor. Menopause was the final, incurable ill, the "death of the woman in the woman."

Women's greater susceptibility to TB was seen as proof of the inherent defectiveness of female physiology. Dr. Azell Ames wrote in 1875: "It being beyond doubt that consumption . . . is itself produced by the failure of the [menstrual] function in the forming of girls . . . one has been the parent of the other with interchangeable priority." Actually, as we know today, it is true that consumption may *result* in suspension of the menses. But at that time consumption was blamed on woman's nature and on her reproductive system. When men were consumptive, doctors sought some environmental factor, such as overexposure, to explain the disease. But in popular imagery, consumption was always effeminate: novels of the time usually featured as male consumptives only such "effete" types as poets, artists, and other men "incompetent" for serious masculine pursuits.

The association of TB with innate feminine weakness was strengthened by the fact that TB is accompanied by an erratic emotional pattern in which a person may behave sometimes frenetically, sometimes morbidly. The behavior characteristic for the disease fit expectations about woman's personality, and the

look of the disease suited—and perhaps helped to create—the prevailing standards of female beauty. The
female consumptive did not lose her feminine identity,
she embodied it: the bright eyes, translucent skin, and
red lips were only an extreme of traditional female
beauty. A romantic myth rose up around the figure of
the female consumptive and was reflected in portrai-
ture and literature: for example, in the sweet and tragic
character of Beth, in *Little Women*. Not only were
women seen as sickly—sickness was seen as feminine.

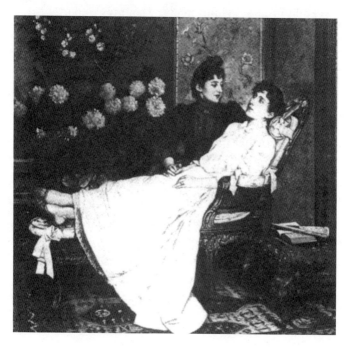

The doctors' view of women as innately sick did not, of course, *make* them sick, or delicate, or idle. But it did provide a powerful rationale against allowing women to act in any other way. Medical arguments were used to explain why women should be barred from medical school (they would faint in anatomy lectures), from higher education altogether, and from voting. For example, a Massachusetts legislator proclaimed:

> Grant suffrage to women, and you will have to build insane asylums in every country, and establish a divorce court in every town. Women are too nervous and hysterical to enter into politics.

Medical arguments seemed to take the malice out of sexual oppression: when you prevented a woman from doing anything active or interesting, you were only doing this for her own good.

THE DOCTORS' STAKE IN WOMEN'S ILLNESS

The myth of female frailty, and the very real cult of female hypochondria that seemed to support the myth, played directly to the financial interests of the medical profession. In the late nineteenth and early twentieth centuries, the "regular" AMA doctors (members of the American Medical Association—the intellectual ancestors of today's doctors) still had no legal monopoly over medical practice and no legal control over the number of people who called themselves "doctors." Competition from lay healers of both sexes, and from what the AMA saw as an excess of formally trained male physicians, had the doctors running scared. A good part of the competition was female: women lay healers and midwives dominated the urban ghettos and the countryside in many areas; suffragists were beating on the doors of the medical schools.

For the doctors, the myth of female frailty thus served two purposes. It helped them to disqualify women as healers, and, of course, it made women highly qualified as patients.* In 1900 there were 173 doctors (engaged in primary patient care) per 100,000 population, compared to 50 per 100,000 today. So, it was in the interests of doctors to cultivate the illnesses of their patients with frequent home visits and drawn-out "treatments." A few dozen well-heeled lady customers were all that a doctor needed for a successful urban practice. Women—at least, women whose husbands could pay the bills—became a natural "client caste" to the developing medical profession.

*See *Witches, Midwives and Nurses* by Barbara Ehrenreich and Deirdre English, 2nd ed. (New York: Feminist Press, 2010).

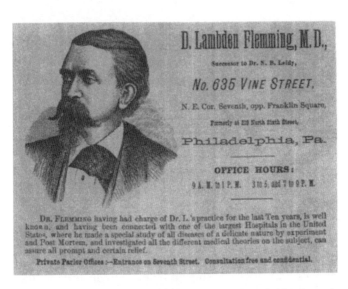

Competition between doctors led them to run ads like this one (from 1878) in the newspapers.

In many ways, the upper-middle-class woman was the ideal patient: her illnesses—and her husband's bank account—seemed almost inexhaustible. Furthermore, she was usually submissive and obedient to the "doctor's orders." The famous Philadelphia doctor S. Weir Mitchell expressed his profession's deep appreciation of the female invalid in 1888:

> With all her weakness, her unstable emotionality, her tendency to morally warp when long nervously ill, she is then far easier to deal with, far more amenable to reason, far more sure to

be comfortable as a patient, than the man who is relatively in a like position. The reasons for this are too obvious to delay me here, and physicians accustomed to deal with both sexes as sick people will be apt to justify my position.

In Mitchell's mind women were not only easier to relate to, but sickness was the very key to femininity: "The man who does not know sick women does not know women."

Some women were quick to place at least some of the blame for female invalidism on the doctors' interests. Dr. Elizabeth Garrett Anderson, an American woman doctor, argued that the extent of female invalidism was much exaggerated by male doctors and that women's natural functions were not really all that debilitating. In the working classes, she observed, work went on during menstruation "without intermission, and, as a rule, without ill effects." (Of course, working-class women could not have afforded the costly medical attention required for female invalidism.) Mary Livermore, a women's suffrage worker, spoke against "the monstrous assumption that woman is a natural invalid," and denounced "the unclean army of 'gynecologists' who seem desirous to convince women that they possess but one set of organs—and that these are always diseased." And Dr. Mary Putnam Jacobi put the matter most forcefully when she wrote in 1895, "I think, finally, it is in the increased attention paid to women, and especially in their new function as lucrative patients, scarcely imagined a hundred years ago, that we find explanation for much of the ill-health among women, freshly discovered today. . . ."

THE "SCIENTIFIC" EXPLANATION
OF FEMALE FRAILTY

As a businessman, the doctor had a direct interest in a social role for women that encouraged them to be

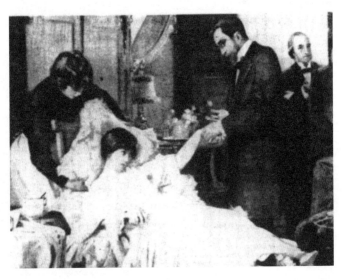

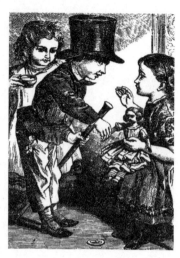

Playing doctor

sick; as a doctor, he had an obligation to find the causes of female complaints. The result was that, as a "scientist," he ended up proposing medical theories that were actually justifications of women's social role.

This was easy enough to do at the time: no one had a very clear idea of human physiology. American medical education, even at the best schools, put few constraints on the doctors' imaginations, offering only a scant introduction to what was known of physiology and anatomy and no training in rigorous scientific method. So doctors had considerable intellectual license to devise whatever theories seemed socially appropriate.

Generally, they traced female disorders either to

women's inherent "defectiveness" or to any sort of activity beyond the mildest "feminine" pursuits—especially sexual, athletic, and mental activity. Thus promiscuity, dancing in hot rooms, and subjection to an overly romantic husband were given as the origins of illness, along with too much reading, too much seriousness or ambition, and worrying.

The underlying medical theory of women's weakness rested on what doctors considered the most basic physiological law: "conservation of energy." According to the first postulate of this theory, each human body contained a set quantity of energy that was directed variously from one organ or function to another. This meant that you could develop one organ or ability only at the expense of others, drawing energy away from the parts not being developed. In particular, the sexual organs competed with the other organs for the body's fixed supply of vital energy. The second postulate of this theory—that reproductivity was central to a woman's biological life—made this competition highly unequal, with the reproductive organs in almost total command of the whole woman.

The implications of the "conservation of energy" theory for male and female roles are important. Let's consider them.

Curiously, from a scientific perspective, *men* didn't jeopardize their reproductivity by engaging in intellectual pursuits. On the contrary, since the mission of upper- and upper-middle-class men was to be doers, not breeders, they had to be careful not to let sex drain energy away from their "higher functions." Doctors warned men not to "spend their seed" (i.e., the essence of their energy) recklessly, but to conserve themselves for the "civilizing endeavors" they were embarked

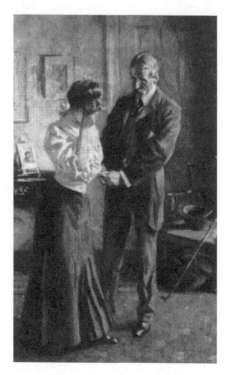

upon. College youths were jealously segregated from women—except on rare sexual sprees in town—and virginity was often prized in men as well as women. Debilitated sperm would result from too much "indulgence," and this in turn could produce "runts," feeble infants, and girls.

On the other hand, because reproduction was woman's grand purpose in life, doctors agreed that women ought to concentrate their physical energy internally, toward the womb. All other activity should be slowed down or stopped during the peak periods of sexual energy use. At the onset of menstruation, women were told to take a great deal of bed rest in order to help focus their strength on regulating their periods—though this might take years. The more time a pregnant woman spent lying down quietly, the better. At menopause, women were often put to bed again.

Doctors and educators were quick to draw the obvious conclusion that, for women, higher education could be physically dangerous. Too much development of the brain, they counseled, would atrophy the uterus. Reproductive development was totally antagonistic to mental development. In a work entitled *Concerning the Physiological and Intellectual Weakness of Women,* the German scientist P. Moebius wrote:

> If we wish woman to fulfill the task of mother-
> hood fully she cannot possess a masculine brain.
> If the feminine abilities were developed to the
> same degree as those of the male, her material
> organs would suffer and we should have before us
> a repulsive and useless hybrid.

In the United States this thesis was set forth most cogently by Dr. Edward Clarke of Harvard College. He warned, in his influential book *Sex in Education* (1873), that higher education was *already* destroying the reproductive abilities of American women.

Even if a woman should choose to devote herself to intellectual or other "unwomanly" pursuits, she could hardly hope to escape the domination of her uterus and ovaries. In *The Diseases of Women* (1849), Dr. F. Hollick wrote: "The Uterus, it must be remembered, is the *controlling* organ in the female body, being the most excitable of all, and so intimately connected, by the ramifications of its numerous nerves, with every other part." To other medical theorists, it was the ovaries that occupied center stage. This passage, written in 1870 by Dr. W. W. Bliss, is, if somewhat overwrought, nonetheless typical:

> Accepting, then these views of the gigantic
> power and influence of the ovaries over the whole

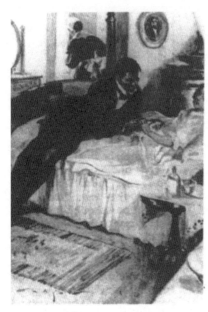

A visit to the invalid

animal economy of woman,—that they are the
most powerful agents in all the commotions of
her system; that on them rest her intellectual
standing in society, her physical perfection, and
all that lends beauty to those fine and delicate
contours which are constant objects of admira-
tion, all that is great, noble and beautiful, all that
is voluptuous, tender, and endearing; that her
fidelity, her devotedness, her perpetual vigilance,
forecast, and all those qualities of mind and dis-
position which inspire respect and love and fit
her as the safest counsellor and friend of man,

spring from the ovaries,—*what must be their influ-ence and power over the great vocation of woman and the august purposes of her existence when these organs have become compromised through disease!* Can the record of woman's mission on earth be otherwise than filled with tales of sorrow, sufferings, and manifold infirmities, all through the influence of these important organs?

This was not mere textbook rhetoric. In their actual medical practices, doctors found uterine and ovarian "disorders" behind almost every female complaint, from headaches to sore throats and indigestion. Curvature of the spine, bad posture, or pains anywhere in the lower half of the body could be the result of "displacement" of the womb, and one doctor ingeniously explained how constipation results from the pressure of the uterus on the rectum. Dr. M. E. Dirix wrote in 1869:

Thus, women are treated for diseases of the stomach, liver, kidneys, heart, lungs, etc.; yet, in most instances, these diseases will be found, on due investigation, to be, in reality, no diseases at all, but merely the sympathetic reactions or the symptoms of one disease, namely, a disease of the womb.

THE PSYCHOLOGY OF THE OVARY

If the uterus and ovaries could dominate woman's entire body, it was only a short step to the ovarian takeover of woman's entire personality. The basic idea, in the nineteenth century, was that female psychology functioned merely as an extension of female reproductivity, and that woman's nature was determined solely by her reproductive functions. The typical medical view was that "the ovaries . . . give to woman all her characteristic of body and mind. . . ." And Dr. Bliss remarked, somewhat spitefully, "The influence of the ovaries over the mind is displayed in woman's artfulness and dissimulation." According to this "psychology of the ovary," all woman's "natural" characteristics were directed from the ovaries, and any abnormalities—from irritability to insanity—could be attributed to some ovarian disease. As one doctor wrote, "All the various and manifold derangements of the reproductive system, peculiar to females, add to the causes of insanity." Conversely, actual physical reproductive problems and diseases, including cancer, could be traced to bad habits and attitudes.

Masturbation was seen as a particularly vicious character defect that led to physical damage, and although this was believed to be true for both men and

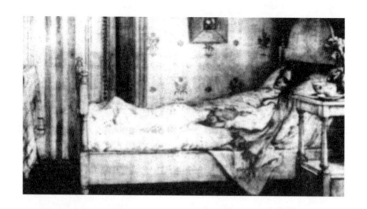

women, doctors seemed more alarmed by female masturbation. They warned that "The Vice" could lead to
menstrual dysfunction, uterine disease, and lesions on
the genitals. Masturbation was one form of "hypersexuality," which was said to lead to consumption; in
turn, consumption might result in hypersexuality. The
association between "hypersexuality" and TB was easily "demonstrated" by pointing to the high rates of
TB among prostitutes. All this fueled the notion that
"sexual disorders" led to disease, and conversely, that
disease lay behind women's sexual desires.

The medical model of female nature, embodied in
the "psychology of the ovary," drew a rigid distinction
between reproductivity and sexuality. Women were
urged by the health books and the doctors to indulge
in deep preoccupation with themselves as "The Sex";

they were to devote themselves to developing their reproductive powers, their maternal instincts, their "femininity." Yet they were told that they had no "natural" sexual feelings whatsoever. They were believed to be completely governed by their ovaries and uteruses, but to be repelled by the sex act itself. In fact, sexual feelings were seen as unwomanly, pathological, and possibly detrimental to the supreme function of reproduction. (Men, on the other hand, *were* believed to have sexual feelings, and many doctors went so far as to condone prostitution on the grounds that the lust of upper-middle-class males should have some outlet other than their delicate wives.)

The doctors themselves never seemed entirely convinced of this view of female nature. While they denied the existence of female sexuality as vigorously as any other men of their times, they were always on the lookout for it. Medically, this vigilance was justified by the idea that female sexuality could only be pathological. So it was only natural for some doctors to test for it by stroking the breasts or the clitoris. But under the stern disapproval, there always lurked the age-old fear of and fascination with woman's "insatiable lust" that, once awakened, might be totally uncontrollable. In 1853, when he was only twenty-five years old, the British physician Robert Brundenell Carter wrote (in a work entitled *On the Pathology and Treatment of Hysteria*):

> ... no one who has realized the amount of moral evil wrought in girls . . . whose prurient desires have been increased by Indian hemp and partially gratified by medical manipulations, can deny that remedy is worse than disease. I have . . . seen young unmarried women, of the middle class of society, reduced by the constant use of the speculum to the mental and moral condition of prostitutes; seeking to give themselves the same indulgence by the practice of solitary vice; and asking every medical practitioner . . . to institute an examination of the sexual organs.

(Did Dr. Carter's patients actually smoke "Indian hemp" or beg for internal examinations? Unfortunately, we have no other authority on the subject than Dr. Carter himself.)

MEDICAL TREATMENTS

Uninformed by anything that we would recognize today as a scientific description of the way human bodies work, the actual practice of medicine at the turn of the century was largely a matter of guesswork, consisting mainly of ancient remedies and occasional daring experiments. Not until 1912, according to one medical estimate, did the average patient, seeking help from the average American doctor, have more than a fifty-fifty chance of benefiting from the encounter. In fact, the average patient ran a significant risk of actually getting worse as a result: bleeding, violent purges, heavy doses of mercury-based drugs, and even opium were standard therapeutic approaches throughout the nineteenth century, for male as well as female patients. Even well into the twentieth century, there was little that we would recognize as modern medical technology. Surgery was still a highly risky enterprise; there were no antibiotics or other "wonder drugs"; and little was understood, medically, of the relationship between nutrition and health or of the role of hormones in regulating physiological processes.

Every patient suffered from this kind of hit-or-miss treatment, but some of the treatments applied to women now seem particularly useless and bizarre. For example, a doctor confronted with what he believed was an inflammation of the reproductive organs might try to "draw away" the inflammation by creating what he thought were counter-irritations—blister or sores on the groin or the thighs. The common medical practice of bleeding by means of leeches also took on some very peculiar forms in the hands of gynecologists. Dr. F. Hollick, speaking of methods of curing amenorrhea (chronic lack of menstrual periods), commented: "Some authors speak very highly of the good effects of leeches, applied to the external lips [of the genitals], a few days before the period is expected." Leeches on the breasts might prove effective too, he observed, because of the deep sympathy between the sexual organs. In some cases leeches were even applied to the cervix despite the danger of their occasional loss in the uterus. (So far as we know, no doctor ever considered perpetrating similar medical insults to the male organs.)

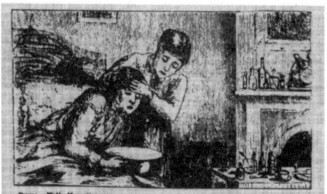

Nurse.—Well, Mrs. Fogy, the Doctor's Ipecac vomits you splendidly. We will soon give you the Calomel and Jalap, next the Castor Oil, then an injection, and after that we will apply the blister and the leeches, and if necessary shave your head. You will be well in three or four weeks,—a little salivated, perhaps, but that's nothing. The Doctor won't charge you more than $40 or $50.

Such methods could be dismissed as well intentioned, if somewhat prurient, experimentation in an age of deep medical ignorance. But there were other "treatments" that were far more sinister—those aimed at altering female *behavior*. The least physically destructive of these was based, simply, on isolation and uninterrupted rest. This was used to treat a host of problems diagnosed as "nervous disorders."

Passivity was the main prescription, along with warm baths, cool baths, abstinence from animal foods and spices, and indulgence in milk and puddings, cereals, and "mild sub-acid fruits." Women were to have a nurse—not a relative—to care for them, to receive no visitors, and as Dr. Dirix wrote, "all sources of mental excitement should be perseveringly guarded against." Charlotte Perkins Gilman was prescribed this type of treatment by Dr. S. Weir Mitchell, who advised her to put away all her pens and books. Gilman later described the experience in the story *The Yellow Wall-Paper*, in which the heroine, a would-be writer, is ordered by her physician-husband to "rest":

> So I take phosphates or phosphites—whichever it is, and tonics and journeys, and air, and exercise, and am absolutely forbidden to "work" until I am well again.

Personally, I disagree with their ideas. Personally, I believe that congenial work, with excitement and change, would do me good.

But what is one to do?

I did write for a while—in spite of them; but it *does* exhaust me a good deal—having to be so sly about it, . . . or else meet with heavy opposition.

Slowly Gilman's heroine begins to lose her grip ("It is getting to be a great effort for me to think straight. Just this nervous weakness, I suppose") and finally she frees herself from her prison—into madness, crawling in endless circles about her room, muttering about the wallpaper.

But it was the field of gynecological surgery that provided the most brutally direct medical treatments of female "personality disorders." And the surgical approach to female psychological problems had what was considered a solid theoretical basis in the theory of the "psychology of the ovary." After all, if a woman's entire personality was dominated by her reproductive organs, then gynecological surgery was the most logical approach to any female psychological problem. Beginning in the late 1860s, doctors began to act on this principle.

At least one of their treatments probably *was*

effective: surgical removal of the clitoris as a cure for sexual arousal. A medical book of this period stated: "Unnatural growth of the clitoris . . . is likely to lead to immorality as well as to serious disease . . . amputation may be necessary." Although many doctors frowned on the practice of removing the clitoris, they tended to agree that this might be necessary in cases of "nymphomania." (The last clitorectomy we know of in the United States was performed twenty-five years ago on a child of five, as a cure for masturbation.)

More widely practiced was the surgical removal of the ovaries—ovariotomy, or "female castration." Thousands of these operations were performed from 1860 to 1890. In his article "The Spermatic Economy," Ben Barker-Benfield describes the invention of the "normal ovariotomy," or removal of ovaries for non-ovarian conditions—in 1872 by Dr. Robert Battey of Rome, Georgia.

> Among the indications were a troublesomeness, eating like a ploughman, masturbation, attempted suicide, erotic tendencies, persecution mania, simple "cussedness," and dysmenorrhea. Most apparent in the enormous variety of symptoms doctors took to indicate castration was a strong current of sexual appetitiveness on the part of women.

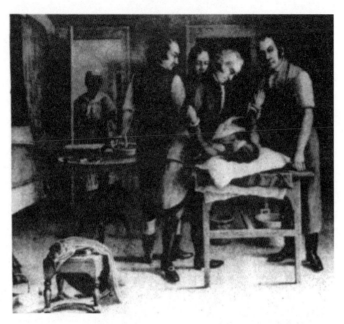

An early nineteenth-century ovariotomy

Patients were often brought in by their husbands, who complained of their unruly behavior. When returned to their husbands, "castrated," they were "tractable, orderly, industrious, and cleanly," according to Dr. Battey. (Today ovariotomy, accompanying a hysterectomy, for example, is not known to have these effects on the personality. One can only wonder what, if any, personality changes Dr. Battey's patients really went through.) Whatever the effects, some doctors claimed to have removed from fifteen hundred to two thousand ovaries; in Barker-Benfield's words, they "handed them around at medical society meetings on plates like trophies."

We could go on cataloging the ludicrous theories, the lurid cures, but the point should be clear: late nineteenth-century medical treatment of women made very little sense as *medicine*, but it was undoubtedly effective at keeping certain women—those who could afford to be patients—in their place. As we have seen, surgery was often performed with the explicit goal of

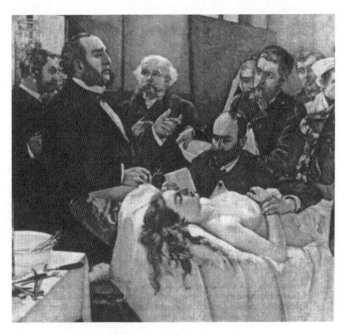

"taming" a high-strung woman, and whether or not the surgery itself was effective, the very threat of surgery was probably enough to bring many women into line. Prescribed bed rest was obviously little more than a kind of benign imprisonment—and the prescriptions prohibiting intellectual activity speak for themselves!

But these are just the extreme "cures." The great majority of upper-middle-class women were never subjected to gynecological surgery or long-term bed rest, yet they too were victims of the prevailing assumptions about women's "weakness" and the necessity of frequent medical attention. The more the doctors "treated," the more they lured women into seeing themselves as sick. The entire mystique of female sickness—the house calls, the tonics and medicines, the health spas—served, above all, to keep a great many women busy at the task of doing nothing. Even among middle-class women who could not afford constant medical attention and who did not have the leisure for full-time invalidism, the myth of female frailty took its toll, with cheap (and often dangerous) patent medicines taking the place of high-priced professional "cures."

One very important effect of all this was a great increase in the upper-middle-class woman's dependence on men. To be sure, the leisured lady of the "better" classes was already financially dependent on her husband. But the cult of invalidism made her seem dependent for her very physical survival on both her doctor and her husband. She might be tired of being a kept woman, she might yearn for a life of meaning and activity, but if she was convinced that she was seriously sick or in danger of becoming so, would she dare to break away? How could she even survive on her own, without the expensive medical care paid for by her husband? Ultimately, she might even become convinced that her restlessness was itself "sick"—just further proof of her need for a confined, inactive life. And if she did overcome the paralyzing assumption of women's innate sickness and begin to act in unconventional ways, a doctor could always be found to prescribe a return to what was considered normal.

In fact, the medical attention directed at these women amounted to what may have been a very effective surveillance system. Doctors were in a position to detect the first signs of rebelliousness, and to interpret them as symptoms of a "disease" which had to be "cured."

SUBVERTING THE SICK ROLE

It would be a mistake to assume that women were merely the passive victims of a medical reign of ter-

Advertisement for a patent medicine

ror. In some ways, they were able to turn the sick role to their own advantage, especially as a form of birth control. For the "well-bred" woman to whom sex really *was* repugnant, and yet a "duty," or for any woman who wanted to avoid pregnancy, "feeling sick" was a way out—and there were few others. Contraceptive methods were virtually unavailable; abortion was risky and illegal. It would never have entered a respectable doctor's head to advise a lady on contraception (if he *had* any advice to offer, which is unlikely). Or to offer to perform an abortion (at least according to AMA propaganda). In fact, doctors devoted considerable energy to "proving" that contraception and abortion were inherently unhealthy, and capable of causing such diseases as cancer. (This was before the pill!) But a doctor *could* help a woman by supporting her claims to be too sick for sex: he could recommend abstinence. So who knows how many of this period's drooping consumptives and listless invalids were actually well women, feigning illness to escape intercourse and pregnancy?

If some women resorted to sickness as a means of birth—and sex—control, others undoubtedly used it to gain attention and a limited measure of power within their families. Today, everybody is familiar with

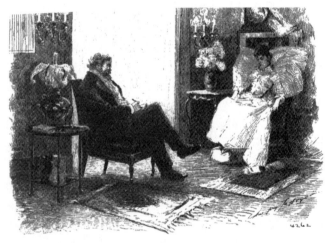

A SOCIETY DISEASE.

Dr. Schmerz. — Nervous prostration. You need rest.
Mrs. Aiken. — Why, I do nothing but rest !
Dr. Schmerz. — Well, try some light employment. Watch other people work.

the (sexist) myth of the mother-in-law whose symptoms conveniently strike during family crises. In the nineteenth century, women developed, in epidemic numbers, an entire syndrome which even doctors sometimes interpreted as a power grab rather than a genuine illness. The new disease was hysteria, which in many ways epitomized the cult of female invalidism. It affected upper- and upper-middle-class women almost exclusively; it has no discernible organic basis; and it was totally resistant to medical treatment. For those reasons alone, it is worth considering in some detail.

A contemporary doctor described the hysterical fit this way:

> The patient . . . loses the ordinary expression of countenance, which is replaced by a vacant stare; becomes agitated; falls before standing; throws her limbs about convulsively; twists the body into all kinds of violent contortions; beats her chest; sometimes tears her hair; and attempts to bite herself and others; and, though a delicate woman, evinces a muscular strength which often requires four or five persons to restrain her effectually.

Hysteria appeared, not only as fits and fainting, but

in every other form: hysterical loss of voice, loss of appetite, hysterical coughing or sneezing, and, of course, hysterical screaming, laughing, and crying. The disease spread wildly, yet almost exclusively in a select clientele of urban middle- and upper-middle-class white women between the ages of fifteen and forty-five.

Doctors became obsessed with this "most, confusing, mysterious and rebellious of diseases." In some ways, it was the ideal disease for the doctors: it was never fatal, and it required an almost endless amount of medical attention. But it was not an ideal disease from the point of view of the husband and family of the afflicted woman. Gentle invalidism had been one thing; violent fits were quite another. So hysteria put the doctors on the spot. It was essential to their professional self-esteem either to find an organic basis for the disease and cure it, or to expose it as a clever charade.

There was plenty of evidence for the latter point of view. With mounting suspicion, the medical literature began to observe that hysterics never had fits when alone, and only when there was something soft to fall on. One doctor accused them of pinning their hair in such a way that it would fall luxuriantly when they fainted. The hysterical "type" began to be charac-

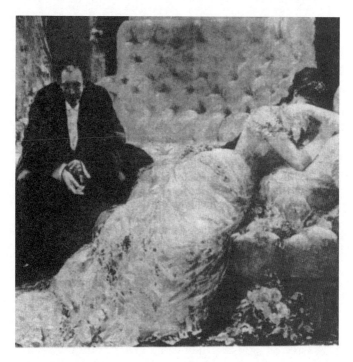

terized as a "petty tyrant" with a "taste for power" over her husband, servants, and children, and, if possible, her doctor.

In historian Carroll Smith-Rosenberg's interpretation, the doctor's accusations had some truth to them: the hysterical fit, for many women, must have been the only acceptable outburst—of rage, of despair, or simply of *energy*—possible. But as a form of revolt it was very limited. No matter how many women might adopt it, it remained completely individualized: hysterics don't unite and fight. As a power play, throwing a fit might give a brief psychological advantage over a husband or a doctor, but ultimately it played into the hands of the doctors by confirming their notion of women as irrational, unpredictable, and diseased.

On the whole, however, doctors did continue to insist that hysteria was a real disease—a disease of the uterus, in fact. (*Hysteria* comes from the Greek word for uterus.) They remained unshaken in their conviction that their own house calls and high physician's fees were absolutely necessary; yet at the same time, in their treatment and in their writing, doctors assumed an increasingly angry and threatening attitude. One doctor wrote, "It will sometimes be advisable to speak in a decided tone, in the presence of the patient, of the necessity of shaving the head, or of giving her a cold shower bath, should she not be soon relieved." He then gave a "scientific" rationalization for this treatment by saying, "The sedative influence of fear may allay, as I have known it to do, the excitement of the nervous centers. . . ."

Carroll Smith-Rosenberg writes that doctors recommended suffocating hysterical women until their fits stopped, beating them across the face and body with wet towels, and embarrassing them in front of family and friends. She quotes Dr. F. C. Skey: "Ridicule

to a woman of sensitive mind, is a powerful weapon
. . . but there is not an emotion equal to fear and the
threat of personal chastisement. . . .They will listen
to the voice of authority." The more women became
hysterical, the more doctors became punitive toward
the disease; and at the same time, they began to see the
disease everywhere themselves until they were diag-
nosing every independent act by a woman, especially a
women's rights action, as "hysterical."

With hysteria, the cult of female invalidism was
carried to its logical conclusion. Society had assigned
affluent women to a life of confinement and inactiv-
ity, and medicine had justified this assignment by
describing women as innately sick. In the epidemic of

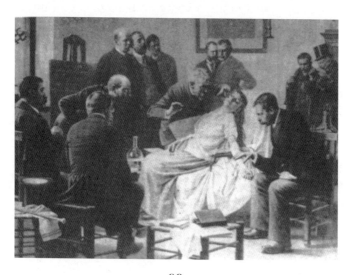

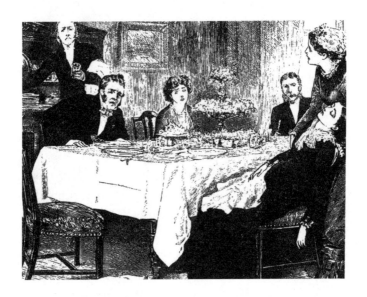

hysteria, women were both accepting their inherent "sickness" *and* finding a way to rebel against an intolerable social role. Sickness, having become a way of life, became a way of rebellion, and medical treatment, which had always had strong overtones of coercion, revealed itself as frankly and brutally repressive.

But hysteria is more than a bizarre twist of medical history. The nineteenth-century epidemic of hysteria had lasting significance because it ushered in a totally new "scientific" approach to the medical management of women.

While the conflict between women and their doctors in America was escalating on the issue of hysteria,

Sigmund Freud, in Vienna, was beginning to work on a treatment that would remove the disease altogether from the arena of gynecology. In one stroke, he solved the problem of hysteria and marked out a new medical specialty. "Psychoanalysis," as Carroll Smith-Rosenberg has said, "is the child of the hysterical woman." Freud's cure was based on changing the rules of the game: in the first place, by eliminating the issue of whether or not the woman was faking. Psychoanalysis, as Thomas Szasz has pointed out, insists that "malingering *is* an illness—in fact, an illness 'more serious' than hysteria." Secondly, Freud established that hysteria was a mental disorder. He banished the traumatic "cures" and legitimized a doctor-patient relationship based solely on talking. His therapy urged the patient to confess her resentments and rebelliousness, and then at last to accept her role as a woman.

Under Freud's influence, the scalpel for the dissection of female nature eventually passed from the gynecologist to the psychiatrist. In some ways, psychoanalysis represented a sharp break with the past and a genuine advance for women: it was not physically injurious, and it did permit women to have sexual feelings (although only vaginal sensations were believed to be normal for adult women; clitoral sensation was "immature" and "masculine"). But in important ways, the Freudian theory of female nature was in direct continuity with the gynecological view which it replaced. It held that the female personality was inherently defective, this time due to the absence of a penis, rather than to the presence of the domineering uterus. Women were still "sick," and their sickness was still totally predestined by their anatomy.

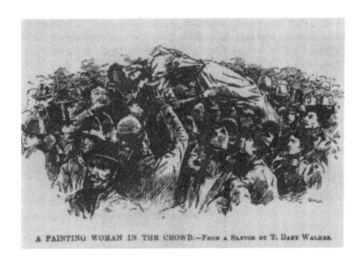

A FAINTING WOMAN IN THE CROWD.—From a Sketch by T. Dart Walker.

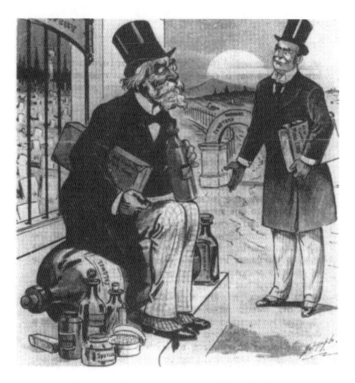

The psychiatrist enters the scene

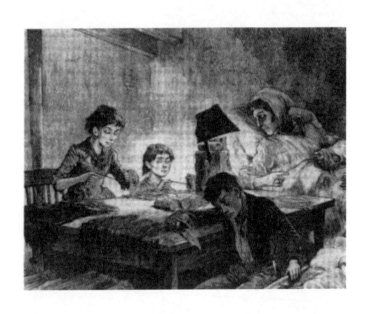

The "Sickening" Women of the Working Class

WHILE DOCTORS WERE MANUFACTURING ILLS FOR affluent women, living conditions in the growing urban slums were making life actually hazardous for poor women. Tenements, which sometimes provided a single privy for dozens of families, were fertile breeding places for typhoid, yellow fever, TB, cholera, and diphtheria. Women who worked outside their homes often put in ten or more hours a day in crowded, poorly ventilated factories or sweatshops, with the constant danger of fatal or disfiguring industrial accidents.

A woman who worked in the garment industry between 1900 and 1920 described her working conditions as follows:

> I see again the dangerously broken stairways in practically all these so-called factories. The win-

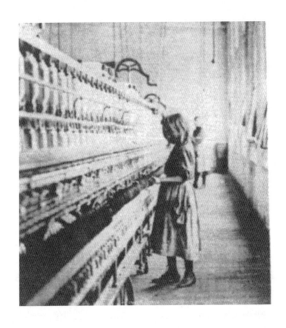

dows few and so dirty that rarely did the sun's rays penetrate these interiors. The wooden floors that were swept once a year. . . . No dressing rooms save the filthy, malodorous lavatory in the dark hall. No fresh drinking water save the cheap soda sold by the poor old peddler. Workshops wherein mice and roaches were as much a part of the physical surroundings as were the machines and the humans. . . .

Sickness, exhaustion, and injury were routine in the life of the working-class woman. Contagious diseases always hit the homes of the poor first and hard-est. Pregnancy, in a fifth- or sixth-floor walk-up flat, really was debilitating, and childbirth, in a crowded tenement room, was often a frantic ordeal. Emma Goldman, who was a trained midwife as well as an anarchist leader, described "the fierce, blind struggle of the women of the poor against frequent pregnan-cies" and told of the agony of seeing children grow up "sickly and undernourished"—if they survived infancy at all. For the woman who labored outside her home, working conditions took an enormous toll. An 1884 report of an investigation of "The Working Girls of Boston," by the Massachusetts Bureau of Statistics of Labor, stated:

> . . . the health of many girls is so poor as to necessitate long rests, one girl being out a year on this account. Another girl in poor health was obliged to leave her work, while one reports that it is not possible for her to work the year round, as she could not stand the strain, not being at all strong. A girl . . . was obliged to leave on account of poor health, being completely run down from badly ventilated work rooms, and obliged to take an eight months rest; she worked a week when not able, but left to save her life. She says she has

to work almost to death to make fair compensation (now $12 per week).

Still, however sick or tired working-class women might have been, they certainly did not have the time or money to support a cult of invalidism. Employers gave no time off for pregnancy or recovery from childbirth, much less for menstrual periods, though the wives of these same employers often retired to bed on all these occasions. A day's absence from work could cost a woman her job, and at home there was

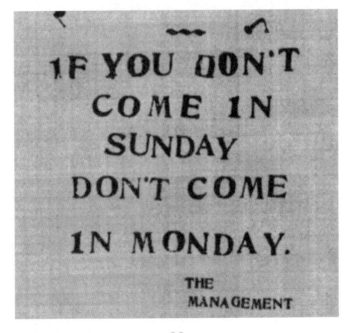

IF YOU DON'T
COME IN
SUNDAY
DON'T COME
IN MONDAY.

THE
MANAGEMENT

no comfortable chaise longue to collapse on while servants managed the household and doctors managed the illness. Two women who worked in the garment industry remembered:

> We only went from bed to work and from work to bed again . . . and sometimes if we sat up a little while at home we were so tired we could not speak to the rest and we hardly knew what we were talking about. And still, there was nothing for us but bed and machine, we could not earn enough to take care of ourselves through the slack season.

Doctors, who zealously indulged the ills of wealthy patients, had no time to spare for the poor. Lillian Wald, a nurse who set up her own practice on New York's Lower East Side, wrote of the troubles she had in finding a doctor to visit a dying woman in the slums. When Emma Goldman asked the doctors she knew whether they had any contraceptive information she could offer the poor, their answers included, "The poor have only themselves to blame; they indulge their appetites too much," and, "When she [the poor woman] uses her brains more, her procreative organs will function less." By and large, medical care for the poor meant home remedies or patent medicines. Only

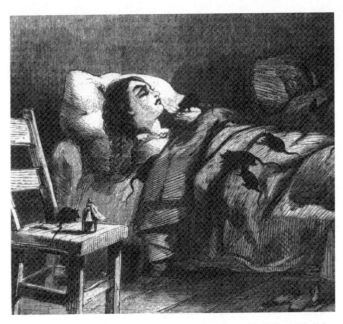

Women's ward in Bellevue Hospital

those too far gone to protest would make the trip to a public hospital where inadequate nursing and unsanitary conditions actually diminished one's chance of survival.

If there was no public outcry about the health of poor women, there was a great deal of upper- and middle-class concern about what the poor were doing to the "health" of the cities.

Americans liked to pride themselves on having a classless society, but there was no way to ignore the fact of increasing class polarization in the cities, where the gracious homes of the affluent were often less than a trolley ride away from such notorious slums as New York's Hell's Kitchen or Lower East Side, or Boston's North Side. There had always been poor people, of course, but there had never been so many of them, and they had never been so visibly different from everyone else. Waves of immigration from southern and eastern Europe had created a working class that had its own distinct languages and customs. By the late nineteenth century immigrant workers outnumbered "native Americans" in the major industrial cities—New York, Cleveland, and Chicago. Cities that had once been peaceably middle class became scenes of epidemics, vice, municipal corruption, and—most frightening of all—riots and violent strikes. The causes of working-

Clinic care for the poor

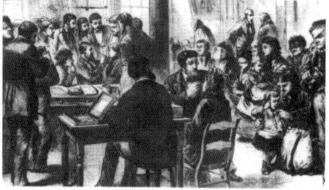

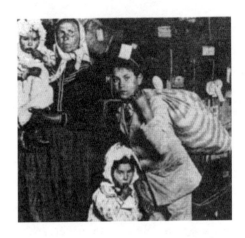

Immigrant family

class unrest were easy enough to see, for anyone who wanted to see them, but it was simpler and more comfortable to blame the poor themselves. As disruption led to repression, and repression fueled new disruptions, wealthier people began to have a sense of being beleaguered in their own land—surrounded by the unwashed, unruly, "un-American" poor.

Class struggle—in the eyes of an increasingly smug and prosperous middle class—was unnatural, un-American, something that only happened "over there" in decadent Europe. Fortunately, "science" provided terms in which class polarization could be talked about without any damage to national pride. The main idea, that the poor were "naturally" inferior, was remarkably parallel to medical theories about women.

First, there was Darwin's theory of evolution, which conveniently hit the popular consciousness in the 1860s and 1870s, just in time to explain the developing class polarization. If some people had more than others—more money, more leisure, better housing, etc.—this was just another case of the workings of that great natural law: the survival of the fittest. It would be "unscientific" to see poverty as the result of social injustice when it was only Nature's way of singling out the manifestly "unfit."

In view of Nature's grand evolutionary purpose, the rebelliousness of the poor was, at best, short-

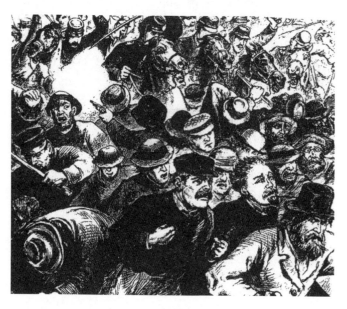

sighted. More commonly, it was seen as an infraction of natural law (i.e., a disease). Contemporary metaphors of class struggle drew as heavily from medicine as from Marx. For example, a writer in a business magazine declared just after the 1886 Haymarket riot that anarchy was a "blood disease" from which, apparently, only Americans of Yankee stock were exempt.

In 1885 a leading minister called for a rational approach to labor unrest, which was fundamentally "physiological" in origin. Race problems came in for the same treatment, the most far-fetched example being Dr. Samuel A. Cartwright's pre-Civil War theory that the tendency of slaves to run away was due to congenital blood disorder—which he dignified with the Latin name "drapetomania" (curable, needless to say, by hard work and whippings). Just as gynecologists found female restlessness to be a symptom of basic ovarian malfunction, so did social observers see the poor as a "race" afflicted with pathological rebellious tendencies.

BIOLOGICAL CLASS WARFARE

Social Darwinism was a comforting ideology for those on top, but it never quite dispelled the fear that, by some irony of natural history, the poor might win

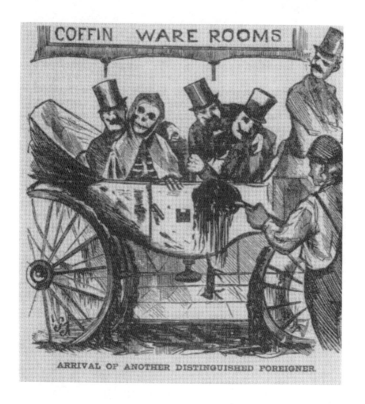

ARRIVAL OF ANOTHER DISTINGUISHED FOREIGNER.

out in the new *biological* class warfare. First, there was the danger of contagion from the poor. Disease was invariably seen as foreign in origin—imported on immigrant ships and bred in immigrant slums. In mid-century, an ex-mayor of New York wrote in his diary that the immigrants were:

> filthy, intemperate, unused to the comforts of life and regardless of its proprieties. . . . [They] flock

to the populous towns of the great west, with disease engendered on shipboard, and increased by bad habits on shore, they inoculate the inhabitants of these beautiful cities.

In her household hygiene book (*Women, Plumbers and Doctors, or Household Sanitation,* 1885) Mrs. H. M. Plunkett warned:

A man may live on the splendid "avenue," in a mansion plumbed in the latest and costliest style, but if, half a mile away, in range with his open window, there is a "slum," or even a neglected tenement house, the zephyrs will come along and pick up the disease germs and bear them onward, distributing them to whomsoever it meets, whether he be a millionaire or a shillingaire, with a perfectly leveling and democratic impartiality.

The germ theory of disease, which became known to the public in the 1890s (in a somewhat distorted fashion), supplied a more concrete basis for class fears about contagion. No longer could abstract "filth," miasmas, or divine will be blamed for disease. There were real, material germs, transmitted by human beings and the objects they touched. Americans, who only a generation ago had feared that bathing was harmful, became preoccupied with germs. The reason people gave for avoiding the ghetto was not the risk of being mugged, but that of being infected with disease. In fact, any public place or object was suspect, as these popular magazine article titles from the period 1900 to 1904 suggest: "Books Spread Contagion," "Contagion by Telephone," "Infection and Postage Stamps," "Disease from Public Laundries," "Menace of the Barber Shop."

There was, certainly, some rational basis for the fear of the poor as a source of contagion. Rates of infectious diseases were higher among the poor, and since scientists themselves were not sure how germs were transmitted, it probably seemed safer just to

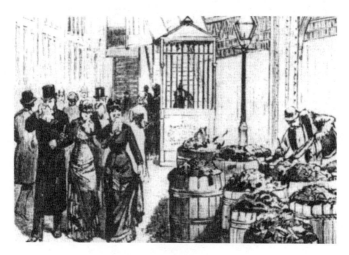

avoid contact with the poor as much as possible. But for our purposes, the distinction between intelligent caution and outright prejudice is not very important. The point is that middle- and upper-class people frequently *expressed* their fear of the poor as a fear of germs, just as white people today might say they don't mind contact with blacks per se; it's crime (or drugs) they're afraid of.

The second front in the biological class warfare featured not germs, but genes. An optimistic reading of Darwin suggested that the "better" class of people would soon outnumber, as well as dominate, the less fit. Poverty was its own cure; epidemic diseases among the poor were the ultimately benign instrument of natural selection. (In the 1870s an observer pointed out that the race problem would soon solve itself. Living in abject poverty in northern cities, freed slaves seemed to be rapidly headed for extinction.) But by the turn of the century it began to seem as if, by some monstrous aberration of natural law, the *better* classes were doomed for extinction.

The birthrate among WASP Americans had been falling since about 1820. Immigrants and blacks, despite their much higher death rates, were believed to breed prolifically. Edward Ross, an early twentieth-century writer who was a liberal for his time, connected the immigrants' fecundity to "their coarse peasant philosophy of sex," "their brawls and their animal pleasures." All this was abhorrent to people of delicacy, but so was the prospect of extinction.

A Professor Edwin Conklin, of Princeton, wrote in the 1890s:

> The cause for alarm is the declining birth rate among the best elements of a population, while it continues to increase among the poorer elements. The descendants of the Puritans and the Cavaliers . . . are already disappearing, and in a few centuries at most, will have given place to more fertile races. . . .

In 1903, President Theodore Roosevelt thundered to the nation the danger of "race suicide":

> Among human beings, as among all other living creatures, if the best specimens do not, and the poorer specimens do, propagate, the type [race] will go down. If Americans of the old stock lead lives of celibate selfishness . . . or if the married are afflicted by that base fear of living which, whether for the sake of themselves or their children forbids them to have more than one or two children, disaster awaits the nation.

He was not against contraception on principle, granting that "doubtless there are communities which it would be in the interest of the world to have die out," but for middle- and upper-class WASP women, it was downright unpatriotic.

THE SPECIAL DANGER OF
WORKING-CLASS WOMEN

As strikers, rioters, or terrorists, working-class men were usually at the forefront of overt political class struggle. Working-class women, on the other hand, were seen as leading the insidious biological warfare. As breeders, they seemed to outdo the delicate or "high-strung" ladies of the better classes. As disease carriers, they were regarded as especially dangerous because they were likely—much more than working-class males—to come into close contact with affluent people. While the men were safely quarantined in heavy industry, the women sought jobs in some of the niches left by leisured females of the middle and upper classes. "Ladies" no longer did their own sewing or housekeeping and were far too well mannered to satisfy their husbands' sexual appetites. So fields such as domestic service, garment manufacture, and prostitution were wide open to working-class women.

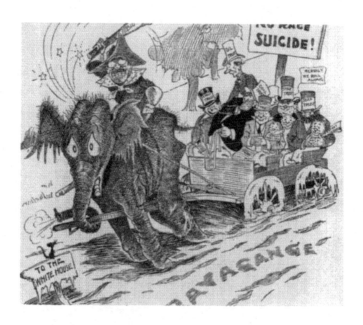

Wherever working-class women, or their products, entered the homes of the "better" classes, could germs be far behind? Garments sewn in tiny tenement sweatshops were suspected of carrying disease germs into wealthy homes, and the garment workers' union played up to this fear by urging people to buy union label clothes because they were made in "hygienic" factories rather than unsupervised tenement shops. The winner of the American Federation of Labor's essay prize of "The Union Label" (c. 1912) wrote: "The union label is, indeed, the only guarantee that the products of any industry are fit to enter decent

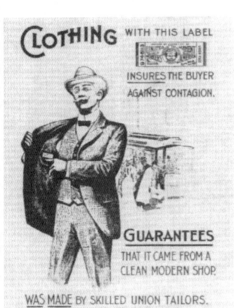

CLOTHING WITH THIS LABEL

INSURES THE BUYER AGAINST CONTAGION.

GUARANTEES

THAT IT CAME FROM A CLEAN MODERN SHOP.

WAS MADE BY SKILLED UNION TAILORS.

SOLD BY ALL FIRST CLASS DEALERS

The picture on the other side REPRESENTS A **TENEMENT HOUSE CIGAR FACTORY.**

BEWARE OF CIGARS MADE IN THOSE FILTHY PLACES.
· **THEY BREED DISEASE** ·

The above Blue Label of the
C.M.I.U. of A.
*on a box containing cigars
is the only safe-guard
against
Tenement House Product.*

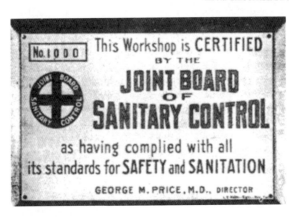

No. 1000 This Workshop is **CERTIFIED**
BY THE
JOINT BOARD
OF
SANITARY CONTROL
as having complied with all
its standards for **SAFETY** and **SANITATION**

GEORGE M. PRICE, M.D., DIRECTOR

112

and cleanly homes." What the union had in mind, of course, was that consumers' interest in hygiene would lead them to support the workers' cause, but this strategy sometimes backfired. AFL President Samuel Gompers complained in 1903 that certain consumer groups composed of "well-meaning philanthropic ladies" were issuing their own labels on the basis of sanitation alone, with no regard for the wages, working conditions, or hours of the women workers, and sometimes even in competition with the workers' own label!

Domestic servants, "the strangers within our gates," were not so easily disposed of. One couldn't do without them, but could one trust them? A survivor of the early decades of the twentieth century told us: "If anything was missing, like a piece of silverware, the servants must have taken it. If anyone in the family got sick, you naturally suspected the servants of carrying something."

The case of "Typhoid Mary" riveted public attention on the dangers of contagion from domestic servants. From a brief account of this case one can appreciate its dramatic impact.

Mary Mallon was an Irish American cook who worked the silk-stocking districts—Oyster Bay, Park Avenue, Sands Point, Dark Harbor, Maine. Her references were good, her employers liked her cooking and were frequently impressed by her steadfastness in the face of family disaster, which seemed to be a routine feature of Ms. Mallon's working life.

When she was finally locked up in 1915, she had left a trail of fifty-two typhoid cases, three of them fatal, in the homes of her employers. Her employers had always tended to blame some other servant in their houses for the typhoid outbreaks, until the relentless detective work of the New York City Health Department exposed Ms. Mallon as the culprit. The lab test proved it: she was a typhoid germ carrier who did not herself suffer from the disease. She was first apprehended in 1907 and placed in solitary quarantine on a tiny island in the East River, then after three years released on parole on the condition that she give up cooking. In 1913 she broke parole and vanished, only to turn up two years later—cooking again—in a Queens hospital struck by typhoid.

Ms. Mallon always insisted that she had never had typhoid fever, was not a typhoid carrier, and was the innocent scapegoat of publicity-hungry health officials. When the health officials came to get her in 1907, she first resisted with a carving fork, then escaped through a back window and barricaded herself with barrels. She was whisked off by car to the public health laboratory with eminent public health authority Dr. Josephine Baker sitting on her chest to subdue her. Her final capture in 1915 was, according to

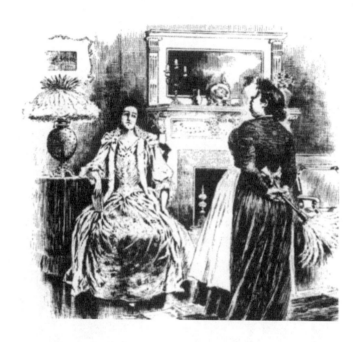

the New York Times, *"nearly as lively as her first one,"*
featuring another chase through windows and backyards.

Here was biological guerrilla warfare at its most virulent. Newspapers' Sunday supplements caricatured
Ms. Mallon as a fiend popping human skulls into a
skillet while the *New York Times* solemnly explained
the dangers of hiring servants without thoroughly
investigating references. Typhoid Mary survived in
folklore as a symbol of the "sickening" woman who
poisons everything she touches.

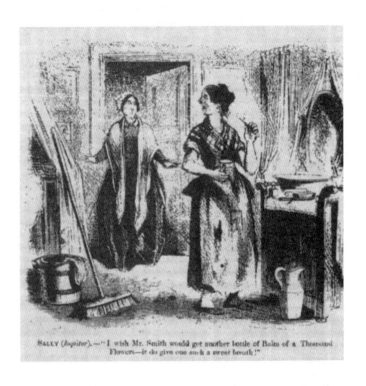

SALLY (loquitur).—" I wish Mr. Smith would get another bottle of Balm of a Thousand Flowers—it do give one such a sweet breath!"

Of course, we now know that, as a typhoid carrier, she was a medical anomaly, a weird exception. Yet to middle-class people of her day she epitomized the threat that *all* working-class women represented: they might *look* innocently robust and healthy, but who knew, finally, what dread disease they harbored.

PROSTITUTES AND VENEREAL DISEASE

Although servants and working-class women in general were all faintly suspect, no one excited middle-class germ fears like the prostitute. Prostitution represented a reservoir of hideous disease, perpetually spilling over into the families of decent people: infecting the fetus in the womb, crippling innocent wives, and dragging the erring males to ruin. Prostitution had not been a problem in the nation's youth, but urbanization and poverty made it a booming industry

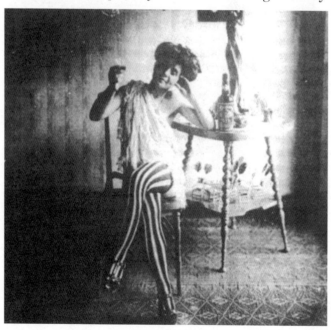

in the late nineteenth and early twentieth centuries. To reform-minded citizens (many of them women's rights activists), prostitution was much more than a public health problem, it was *the* Social Evil, underlying municipal corruption, family breakdown in the lower classes, and public immorality in general.

Some of the best data we have on the extent of prostitution and VD during the first decades of the century comes from a series of studies sponsored by

Police raid on a brothel

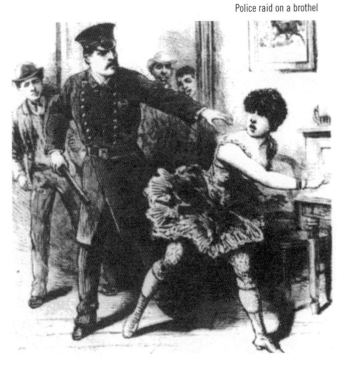

John D. Rockefeller Jr.'s Bureau of Social Hygiene (a private, voluntary agency). According to one of the Bureau reports, prepared by Dr. Howard Woolston, alarm reached a peak in the 1910s when the prospect of US involvement in the First World War "brought home to the American people as nothing in our previous history had ever done, the menace of prostitution and venereal diseases to the young manhood of our country."

By 1917 (the date of this report), police efforts had already cut severely into the trade, and yet Dr. Woolston found two hundred thousand women "in the regular army of vice," an estimated 60 to 75 percent of them carrying VD. As a result, an estimated 25 to 35 percent of the adult urban population were infected. Not only laboring men with their "animal pleasures," but also businessmen, college boys, and professional men were among the victims.

Only the most enlightened—feminists and social reformers—traced prostitution to poverty and oppressive sex roles. Moralists blamed "male lust and female frailty." More "scientific" observers blamed the prostitute herself or, rather, her "congenital defects." In the 1917 study Dr. Woolston went out of his way to discount economic motivations in prostitutes, and seriously concluded that "the ordinary prostitute appears to be a short, stocky woman." Further, at least one-third of them were mentally defective:

> It is a well-known fact that feeblemindedness is hereditary. Consequently, some of the mental anomalies of the prostitutes can be directly traced to weakness in the stock from which they come. . . . In 297 of the 1,000 families [of prostitutes surveyed] . . . some actively vicious or clearly recognized degenerate strain was known to be present. It is likely that a more complete investigation would have revealed an even larger number.

However, prostitutes were not seen as a breed apart from the average working-class woman. Dr. Woolston and other surveyors found that there was considerable shuttling back and forth between prostitution and low-paid jobs such as domestic service. In the popular imagination, working-class women were all somewhat sickening, whether because they spread diseases or dragged down the "race" with their inferior and all-too-plentiful offspring. If the upper-middle-class woman had health problems, the working-class woman *was* a health problem. Not for her the domineering and indulgent physician; for her there was the public health officer.

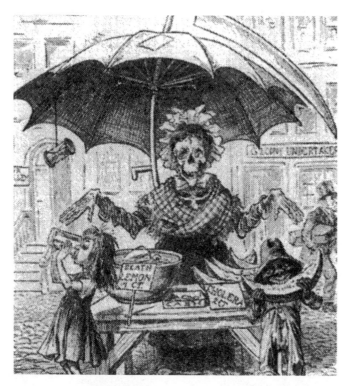

Death posing as a female peddler in the slums of New York (1882)

THE MIDDLE-CLASS OFFENSIVE:
PUBLIC HEALTH

Beginning in the last decades of the nineteenth century, the "better" classes launched an organized political offensive against poor and working people. There were repressive anti-labor measures, civic "reforms" aimed at reducing the electoral power of immigrant groups, and, later, laws to stop the immigration of Italians, Jews, Poles, and other "inferior" races. In the *biological* class warfare, the two major middle-class thrusts were the public health movement and the birth

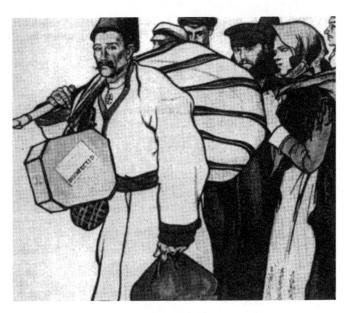

control movement, directed against the twin threats of contagion and "out breeding," respectively. Both of these movements drew heavily on the energies of middle- and upper-middle-class women who, as our historical period wore on, were becoming increasingly dissatisfied with the life of enforced leisure.

The progressive achievements of these movements are obvious: legal contraception, free garbage removal, compulsory immunization, to name just a few. But their story as social movements is somewhat more ambiguous: both mobilized large numbers of middle- and upper-class women in a way which solidified their new relationship to working-class women— not as sisters, but as *uplifters*.

The public health movement had an evangelical tone which put it in the same moral league with the temperance and "social purity" (anti-prostitution) movements. In fact, the distinction between "dirt" and "sin" was still unclear. An earlier generation had traced all disease to immorality and relied on prayer rather than sanitation to ward off epidemics. The sin theory of disease provided a comforting explanation of why epidemics were most virulent in the areas inhabited by "vicious, intemperate, and atheistic" immigrant workers. But the theory was not so comforting when it became clear that epidemics could also carry off bankers, ministers, and society ladies. The blame shifted from sin to "dirt," but the moral implications hardly changed. Typhoid epidemics, according to the household hygiene book we cited earlier, had been looked upon as "chastening visitations of God for moral delinquencies," but, in the light of contemporary sanitary "science," were recognized as "the strict adjustments of penalty for His broken physical laws." Dr. Elizabeth Blackwell called sanitation "the *reverential* acceptance of the *divine* laws of health" (emphasis added).

The moral aspect of public health was also reflected in its strong bureaucratic ties to the police. In New York City, which set the pattern for public health administration in other cities, public health was originally a police function, and the first Metropolitan Board of Health included equal numbers of doctors and police officials. The association between public health and police functions (crime and disease) was strengthened by the realization in the latter part of the first decade of the twentieth century that people—not books, coins, or breezes—were the main carriers of disease. Then public health officers began to take on police functions themselves, tracking down and quarantining (as in the case of Typhoid Mary) characters suspected of spreading disease. The

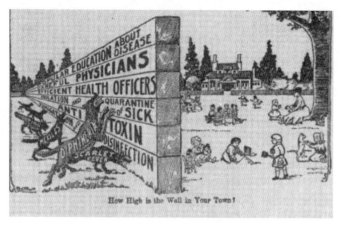

How High is the Wall in Your Town?

Public health poster (1910)

crime-fighting zeal of the public health officials comes through clearly in a 1910 article in *The Nation*, calling for public health police powers to hunt down an estimated twenty thousand "loose" TB victims:

> It is as if the enemy had stolen through the pickets at night and there were no police or soldiers to follow them. The tubercle bacilli swarm through the city on silent wings, grimly laughing at the pamphlets and lectures and scattered deeds of charity which they find so easy to elude.

Public health crusaders were perfectly frank about their class interests in reform. The National Association for the Study and Prevention of Tuberculosis pre-

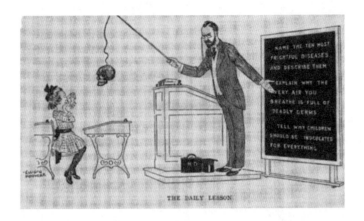

THE DAILY LESSON

sented detailed calculations of the costs of TB among the poor to the middle class—in terms of absenteeism by workers, relief required for orphans, etc. In a more lyrical vein, Mrs. Plunkett, the household hygiene expert, asked how the problem of poverty and disease was to be solved, and answered her own question:

> Through the agency of *enlightened selfishness* . . . the upper 10,000 are learning that their sanitary welfare is indissolubly connected to that of the lower 10 millions, and it is this perception of this truth that has caused the "wave of emotional interest" in the condition of the poorer classes. . . . The class to be elevated resent supervision and care little for health or cleanliness till taught but already some great and definite steps have been taken.

In the war against dirt and germs it was only natural that women should take the lead. Weren't women the divinely appointed sanitation officers of their own homes? In 1881 an American household hygiene book quoted the president of the British Medical Association (at the same time probably more prestigious here than the AMA) as placing almost full responsibility for health on "the character of the presiding genius of the home, or the woman who rules over that small domain." But woman's sanitary responsibilities obviously could not end at her doorstep. In this thesis on nineteenth century "social purity" movements, David Pivar writes:

> Women of the middle class believed in high standards of sanitation and cleanliness and feared the contagions located in the slums and on the streets. Long dresses, dragging the muck, transported dirt, dust and germs into the home. Clothing manufactured in tenement houses found its way into middle class homes. Disease could not be stopped with a closed door. If the home was to be protected, women could not turn inward; they were forced to make the community more "home-like." Only through improvements in public health and morals could the sanctity of the home be assured.

Women doctors entered public health in disproportionate numbers (partly because it was easier for a woman to enter public health than to set up in private practice). At the grassroots level, public health was very much a women's movement (of upper-middle-class women) with close ties to the temperance and suffrage movements.

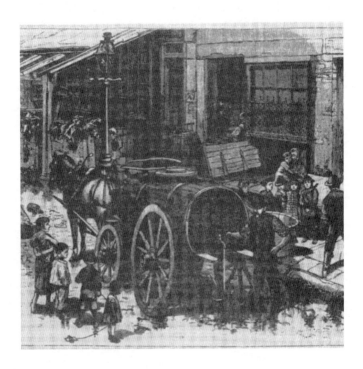

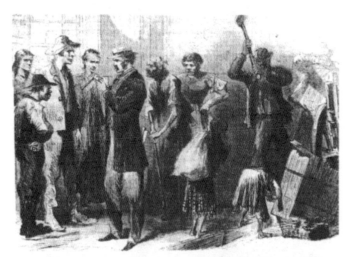

Board of Health raid on a tenement

THE MIDDLE-CLASS OFFENSIVE:
BIRTH CONTROL

Public health was always respectable, but the birth control movement started out in the disreputable company of anarchists, socialists, and extreme feminists. Emma Goldman was jailed for speaking on birth control, and the young Margaret Sanger pushed it in her socialist/feminist journal *The Woman Rebel*. At first, other middle-class reformers saw birth control as a wicked scheme to "take the penalty out of vice," and "degrade the wife to the level of the prostitute."

But as the movement matured under Sanger's single-handed leadership and attracted the support of

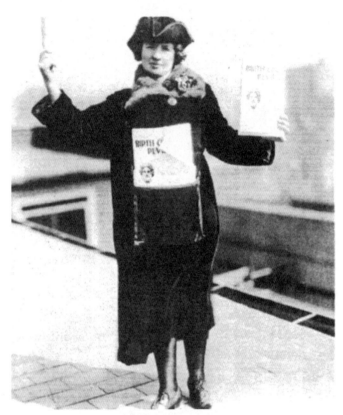

Margaret Sanger selling her *Birth Control Review* in the streets of New York, 1915

thousands of upper-middle- and upper-class women, it began to make a frank appeal to upper-middle-class self-interest. By the late 1910s Sanger was blaming all the problems of the world—war, poverty, prostitution, famine, feeblemindedness—on overpopulation, and she put the blame for overpopulation squarely on women:

> While unknowingly laying the foundations of tyrannies and providing the human tinder for racial conflagrations woman was also unknowingly creating slums, filling asylums with the insane, and institutions with other defectives. She was replenishing the ranks of prostitutes, furnishing grist for the criminal courts and inmates for prisons. Had she planned deliberately to achieve this tragic total of human waste and misery, she could hardly have done it more effectively.

And in case that did not make clear *which* women Sanger blamed, she wrote, in 1918, that "all our problems are the result of overbreeding among the working class."

Birth control offered the possibility of qualitative as well as quantitative control of the population. "More children from the fit, less from the unfit—that is the chief issue of birth control," Sanger declared in 1919. Just who was fit and who was unfit—and how you would impose birth control on one group and keep it away from the other—was not altogether clear. Ms. Sanger usually limited her definition of the "unfit" to the feebleminded (as judged by the newly invented IQ test), but some of her associates in the American Birth Control League were explicitly racist.

Guy Irving Burch, an officer of Sanger's National Committee on Federal Legislation for Birth Control, explained his interest in birth control thus:

> My family on both sides were early colonial and pioneer stock and I have long worked with the American Coalition of Patriotic Societies to prevent the American people from being replaced by alien or Negro stock, whether it be by immigration or by overly high birth rates among others in this country.

Another birth control advocate urged that "to offset the so-called 'yellow peril,'" the United States should, "spread birth control knowledge abroad so as to decrease the quantity of people whose unchecked reproduction threatens international peace."

A few farsighted physicians joined in the campaign to make contraception acceptable to the middle class by pointing out its possibilities for population control. In his 1912 presidential address to the AMA, Dr. Abraham Jacobi endorsed birth control, citing the high fertility of immigrants and the rising cost of welfare. Dr. Robert Dickinson, a gynecologist and one of Sanger's most steadfast medical allies, urged his fellow doctors in 1916 to "take hold of this matter [birth control] and not let it go to the radicals." With the help of men like Dr. Dickinson, Ms. Sanger was able to begin the first birth control services—appropriately enough, in the slums of New York City.

Contraception did not become legal until a 1938 court ruling allowed physicians to import, mail, and prescribe birth control devices. This was a great step forward for women and the credit goes largely to Margaret Sanger's courage and determination.

We want to be clear about our position on this issue. We think birth control should be available on demand for all women, of all classes and ethnic groups. We do not subscribe to the view that birth control is liberating for some women, but "genocidal" for others. What we are criticizing is the line that the birth control movement advanced in order to make its gains. The fact that the birth control movement took a racist and classist line makes even the final victory a dubious one.

But here we must ask ourselves: Could the birth control movement have succeeded any other way, given the context of American society at the time? If the birth control movement had advanced purely feminist arguments for contraception, would it have had the power or influence to succeed? We might ask a similar question about the public health movement: Would there have been any *public health reforms if these had not been in the direct self-interest of wealthy and powerful people? These questions are, of course, unanswerable, but they do point to the fundamental ambiguity of* reform *in an otherwise oppressive society.*

WOMEN "UPLIFT" WOMEN

The public health movement never succeeded in quarantining all the germ-ridden ghetto residents, and the birth control movement fell far short of its goals of race "purification." In fact, public health measures made the cities healthier for the poor as well as for the rich, and birth control, ironically, had its biggest impact on the population of the middle and upper classes themselves. Certainly, we owe a great deal to the masses of women who worked in these two movements, whatever their motivations. The sad thing is that the reform movements served to deepen the division of women along class lines: on the one side were the reformers (middle- and upper-middle-class women), on the other side the objects of reform (working-class women).

The reformers were women who rebelled against the empty leisure required of "ladies." They wanted to *do* something, wanted a project worthy of their untapped moral sensitivities and social concerns. For many, that project became the great task of "uplifting" working-class women. Public health and birth control

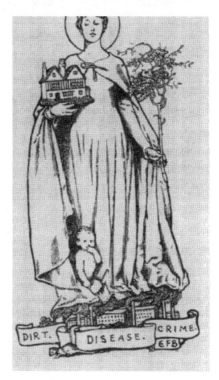

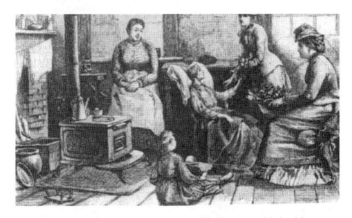

Wealthy women visit the sick poor

were the more impersonal part of the campaign; many women reformers were drawn into direct contact with poor women. Anti-vice crusaders attempted to reform prostitutes; social workers went into the slums to teach the poor home economics and "American values"; clubwomen set up discussion groups on ethical issues for young working women. According to home economics books of the time, even the woman who stayed at home had a missionary responsibility to instruct her servant in moral and sanitary matters and to prepare her to be a "good wife."

The upper-middle-class woman activist of the 1890s and early twentieth century had left her sisters far behind on their chaise longues, in sick rooms and health spas. She had rejected a medical ideology that defined her as sick and confined her to uselessness. But she seems to have won "release" only on condition that she both remain true to the interest of her class and take on social roles that were extensions of the wife/mother role, as social worker or volunteer "uplifter." In these roles, bringing the gospel of hygiene, public health, home economics, etc. to the poor, she was necessarily patronizing, at times antagonistic, in her relations with poor women.

The issue of health—female health and family health—which potentially could have united women of different classes, now divided them into reformers on one side and "problems" on the other. Upper-middle-class women did not turn against the medical profession that had imprisoned them and rejected poor women; they did not unite with poor women to create a movement which could demand a single standard of health and health care for all women. In the public health and birth control movements they allied themselves *with* doctors, against the threats posed by the poor.

However, we do not want to leave the impression that upper-middle-class women were simply "led astray," by ideological considerations, from the task of building a health movement for and with all women. It is true that women

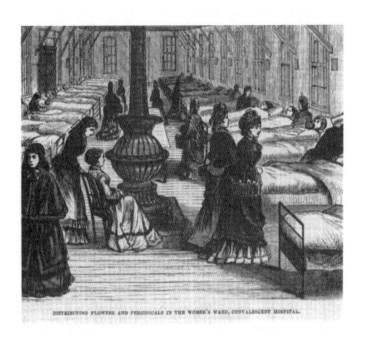

DISTRIBUTING FLOWERS AND PERIODICALS IN THE WOMEN'S WARD, CONVALESCENT HOSPITAL.

of all social groups have a potential unity around common biological experiences. And it is true that medical ideology—in the form of both "scientific" theory and popular beliefs—did its best to deny the commonality of women's experience and to separate women into the sick (or vulnerable) and the sickening (or dangerous). But this ideology would never have been accepted by men—or women—of the upper classes if it hadn't been rooted in economic reality.

In many ways, the situations of women in the classes we have considered were complementary. Upper-middle-

class women would not have had the leisure to be invalids, or reformers, if it had not been for the exploitation of working-class people (including women and children); they would not have been free from household work if it had not been for the labor of domestic servants and the women who worked in factories manufacturing clothes and other household items that had once been made in the home. Medical myths and biological fears did not create the class differences among women; they only gave them "scientific" plausibility.

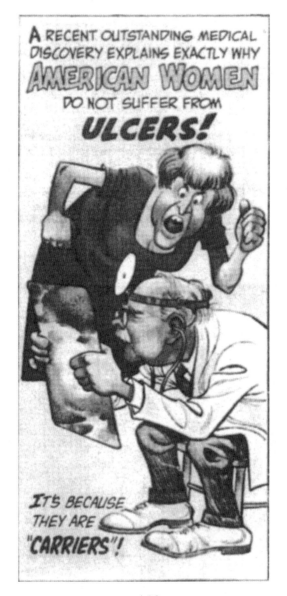

Notes on the Situation Today (1973)

ONE HUNDRED YEARS HAVE PASSED SINCE THE HEY-day of wholesale ovariotomies, hysteria, and enforced invalidism. Medical theory no longer asserts that some women are congenitally sick, while others are potentially sickening. Yet in some important ways, the relationship between women and the medical system has changed very little, if at all.

Middle- and upper-class women are still a "client caste" to the medical profession. For a host of reasons connected with reproductivity women continue to visit doctors and enter hospitals far more frequently than men do. Pregnancy, if no longer described explic-itly as a disease, is still treated like a medical problem, in exactly the same settings and by exactly the same personnel used for the treatment of actual disorders. Childbirth is no longer a cause for lengthy confine-ment, but it is, more so than ever, an alienating, surgical event. Irregular menstruation is no longer viewed as calamitous, but doctors are more than willing to provide costly hormonal "cures." Menopause, while no longer an indication for terminal bed rest, is still described to medical students as "the most serious endocrinological disorder next to diabetes," "curable" of course, with expensive estrogen therapy. And while the rip-roaring frontier days of gynecological surgery may be gone forever, some doctors, such as Robert McCleery, in *One Life, One Physician* (1971), acknowledge that up to half of the hysterectomies performed in the United States (and perhaps a large proportion of radical mastectomies* performed anywhere) are unnecessary.

In fact, women's dependence on doctors (hence doctors' dependence on women) may have increased since 1900. Doctors moved in on each sexual or reproductive right as soon as it was liberated: they now control abortion and almost all reliable means of contraception. Even sexual unresponsiveness—the "natural" condition of our great-grandmothers—has become a medical problem, with its own sex "clinics" and its own brand of medical specialists.

---

*Mastectomy is the surgical removal of the breast. Some mastectomies involve considerable damage to the muscles around the upper arm.

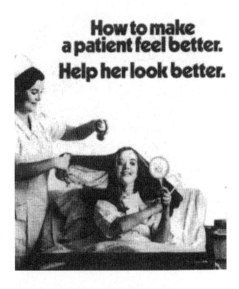

How to make a patient feel better. Help her look better.

There are still profound class differences in women's relationship to the medical system. On the medical marketplace millions of women—far more than the statistically "poor"—cannot afford the most basic, preventive services, never mind the luxury items. The fragmented pattern of public health services for low-income women—here a VD clinic, there a Planned Parenthood clinic, almost nowhere a low-cost comprehensive care center—shows that they are still treated more as public health problems than as human beings needing individualized medical care. For no groups is this truer than for black, Puerto Rican, and Chicana women. Once lumped together with Italians, Poles,

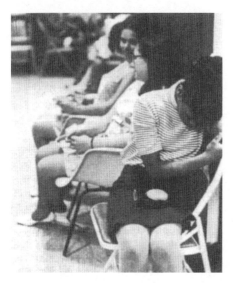

Clinic waiting room

and other immigrant groups as "inferior stock," Third World women now stand almost alone as the special target of such population control measures as involuntary sterilization.

We could go on tracing continuities from the nineteenth and early twentieth centuries, but we are struck even more by the differences. The situation of both doctors and women has changed drastically. For women, even in the upper middle class, the days of total leisure are over. More and more women work outside the home, and, within the home, the servants are gone. The woman who works outside holds down two jobs—that of a paid worker and that of an unpaid housekeeper and mother. Even the more affluent, "leisured" housewife is expected to be healthy and active at all times, able to chauffeur the kids around, manage the house, and perform as a gracious wife and hostess. In a statement that speaks for almost all of us, one working-class housewife told a medical sociologist, "Sometimes I'd like to be sick, but I don't have the time."

Doctors today don't seem to have the time for us to be sick anymore either. In the late nineteenth century there was, by present standards, an excess of doctors in the cities. Competition was fierce, and there was a strong motivation to overtreat ill women and discover illnesses among well women. But in the early 1900s the medical profession won the legal right to control its own numbers—to set standards for medical schools, close "substandard" schools, etc. (See our pamphlet *Witches, Midwives and Nurses* for more on this phase.) The closing of medical schools in the teens and twenties, followed by decades of AMA lobbying against Federal aid to medical schools, eventually produced the familiar doctor shortage. Only a few doctors base their practices on intimate care given to a small number of rich people. Most spread their services fairly thinly over a large number of middle- or working-class people. The result is the ten-minute gynecological appointment, the fifteen-minute annual checkup (these are the actual times allotted in one of the New York area's largest and most reputable group practices), and during such quickie examinations the amount of patient/doctor dialogue is reduced to a minimum.

So for most of us, the intimate, paternalistic doctor-patient relationship of the nineteenth century is little more than a historical curiosity. Being sick is no longer consistent with our social roles nor is it a practical possibility, given the doctor shortage. Our medical image has come almost full circle from the days of female invalidism. Because women have longer life expectancies than men, with lower risks of heart disease, stroke, and lung cancer, *we* are considered the

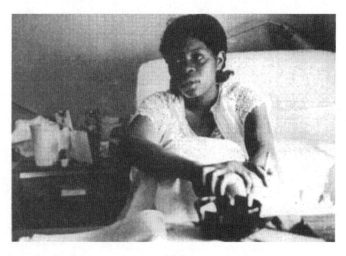

"stronger" sex, and the popular health books eagerly advise us how to keep our *husbands* alive and well. Just as surely as ever, our medical care does serve to enforce our social role, only now that role is to be workers (domestic or otherwise), not pampered invalids.

When a doctor cannot quickly pinpoint the organic cause of a woman's complaint, he is quick to suspect psychosomatic causes (i.e., malingering). A 1973 study written by two doctors, Jean and John Lennane, and published in a prestigious medical journal, concluded:

> Dysmennorhea [menstrual cramps], nausea of pregnancy, pain in labor and infantile behavioral disturbances are conditions commonly considered to be caused or aggravated by psychogenic factors. Although such scientific evidence as exists clearly implicates organic causes, acceptance of a psychogenic origin has led to an irrational and ineffective approach to their management. Because these conditions affect only women, the cloudy thinking that characterizes the relevant literature may be due to a form of sexual prejudice.

The medical profession helped to create the popular notion of women as sickly in the first place: now it seems to have turned around and blamed the victim.

Women patients are seen as silly, self-indulgent, and superstitious. Tranquilizers are used to keep us on the job when no quick medical fix can be found. How many times do we go to a doctor feeling sick and leave, after a diagnosis of "psychosomatic," feeling *crazy*?

In fact, the tendency of doctors to diagnose our complaints as psychosomatic shows that the medical view of women has not really shifted from "sick" to "well"; it has shifted from "physically sick" to "mentally ill." Today it is psychiatry, much more than gynecology, that upholds the sexist tenet of women's fundamental defectiveness. In classical psychoanalytic theory there is no such things as a mentally well woman: the ambitious woman, not content to be a wife and mother, is seen as neurotically rejecting her femininity while the woman who is content to be with her family may be viewed as "infantile." Both are potentially sickening to those around them. The ambitious woman can be blamed for "emasculating" men, and the devoted mother can be blamed for "infecting" her sons with guilt and dependency. One result, as Phyllis Chesler has shown in her book *Women and Madness* (1972), is that women are more likely than men to be incarcerated in mental hospitals.

In general, the mainstream of psychological theory still upholds the view that middle-class women should

"Don't give it a second thought, Miss Watkins. All my patients are crazy about me."

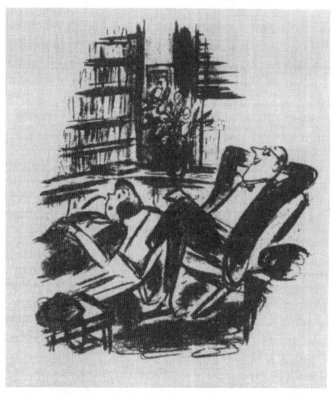

stay at home, but for new reasons. In the past, gynecology justified women's confinement to the home on the basis of women's supposed physical frailty and unfitness for outside pursuits. But now that middle-class women are finally sturdy enough to go out to work, they are being told that their children are too "delicate" to be left behind. Psychology has "discovered" that at least up to the age of three, children are totally dependent on one-to-one mothering! Send your child out to day care or hire a babysitter and you supposedly inflict a risk of lasting neurosis. (Pediatricians

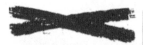

for management of the
emotional "problem patient"

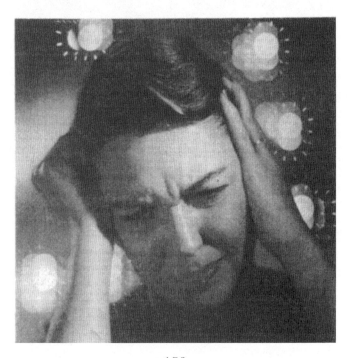

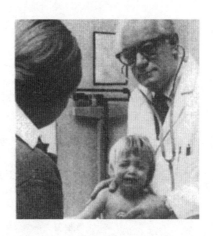

add that day care centers are notorious for spreading infectious diseases.) So now it is the small child of the middle-class woman who has become too "delicate" for the "outside world" of day care, babysitters, and play groups. In contrast, the children of welfare mothers—who *ought* to be out working, according to current moral standards—are emotionally sturdy enough for the most alienating, industrial-style day care centers.

We can only marvel at the endless plasticity of a medical "science" that can adjust its theories for age, sex, or social class, depending on the needs of time. Certainly, science, to *be* science, must change its theories to fit new data. What is amazing about medical "science" as it relates to women is that the theories change so neatly to fit the needs of the dominant, male ideology.

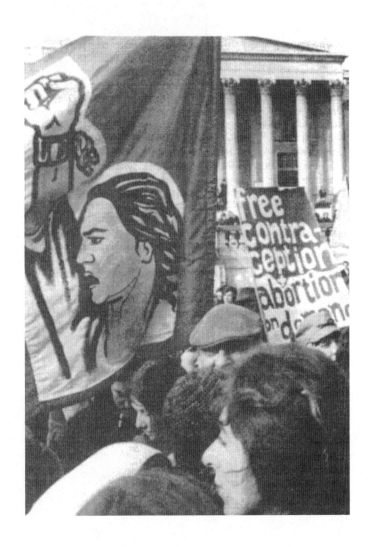

From Here On: Concluding Thoughts

THE MEDICAL SYSTEM IS NOT JUST A SERVICE INDUS-try. It is a powerful instrument of social control, replacing organized religion as a prime source of sexist ideology and an enforcer of sex roles. Certainly, it is not the *only* haven of institutional sexism in our society—the educational system may be equally important or even more important. But it has the unique authority to judge who is sick and who is well, who is fit and who is unfit. The presumed scientific basis of medicine lends credibility to these judgments, yet as we have seen, the judgments themselves have no consistent basis in biology. At one time, women of one class were judged uniformly sick while women of another class were uniformly well though potentially sickening to others. Today we are all well, at least well enough to work; our sickness is "only mental." Our social roles, and not our innate biology, determine our state of

153

health. Medicine does not invent our social roles, it merely interprets them to us as biological destiny.

As feminists we are totally antagonistic to the medical system as a source of sexist ideology. But at the same time, we are totally dependent on medical *technology* for some of the most basic and primitive freedoms we require as women—freedom from unwanted pregnancies, freedom from chronic physical disability. We may be repelled by the crude sexism we encounter in doctors, we may be enraged by the sophisticated sexism passed off as medical theory, but we have nowhere else to turn for abortions, diaphragms, antibiotics, and essential surgery.

Our sheer physical dependence on medical technology makes the medical system all the more powerful as a source of sexist ideology. They have us, so to speak, by the ovaries. All too often, women have humbly accepted the ideological judgments ("you are sick, silly, hysterical, inadequate," etc.) as the price of whatever technological freedoms they could wrest from the system. Now that we have come to take these freedoms just a little bit for granted, we sometimes lean too far the other way—rejecting the technology itself because we cannot stomach the ideological wrapping.

So we seem to be caught in a contradiction: there is something in the medical system that we want, that

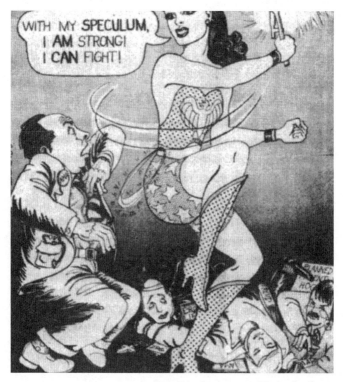

From *Sister*, the newspaper of the Los Angeles Women's Center (July 1973)

we cannot live without, but is there any way to get it on our own terms? When we make demands of the medical system, or of a particular health institution, just what is it that we want? Do we want just "more services"—when every one of them is loaded with a message of oppression? When these services may have little to do with our real needs, and may in fact discount our real needs or substitute medically manufactured needs?

Clearly, our demands must go beyond the merely quantitative. We want more than "more"; we want a new *style*, and we want a new *substance* of medical practice as it relates to women. And yet we must never get so hung up on the ideological niceties that we forget that "more" alone is still crucial—an issue of survival—for millions of women who still lack the most routine care and preventive services, and who cannot function fully as women until they have them.

It is only in the context of our ambivalence to the medical system that we can assess the historic importance of the self-help movement.

Self-help, which emphasizes self-examination and self-knowledge, is an attempt to seize the *technology* without buying the ideology. Self-help has no limits beyond those imposed by our imagination and our resources. It *could* expand far beyond self-examination to include lay (though not untrained) treatment for many common problems—lay prenatal and delivery assistance, lay abortions, and so on. But if our imaginations are unlimited, our resources *are* limited. If we are concerned with the care of *all* women—and not just those with the leisure for self-help enterprises—

for *all* their problems—and not just the uncomplicated disorders of youth—then we are once again up against the medical system with its complex and expensive technology.

In fact, it is in precisely this confrontation that self-help proves its worth. It arms us to demand what we need, not what someone thinks we should get. It gives us a vision of what medical care *could* mean—a system in which needs are not met at the price of dignity.

Self-help is not an alternative to confronting the medical system with the demands for reform of existing institutions. Self-help, or more generally, self-knowledge, is critical to that confrontation.

Health is an issue for women which has the potential to cut across class and race lines. The medical system, more than any other institution of American society, reduces us to a biological category, stripped of our occupations, lifestyles, and individualities. There is very little danger today that middle-class women will relate to poor and working-class women purely as missionaries or "organizers" for health reforms because middle-class women are becoming so acutely aware of their *own* oppression in the medical system. The growth of feminist consciousness gives us the possibility, for the first time, of a truly egalitarian, mass women's health movement.

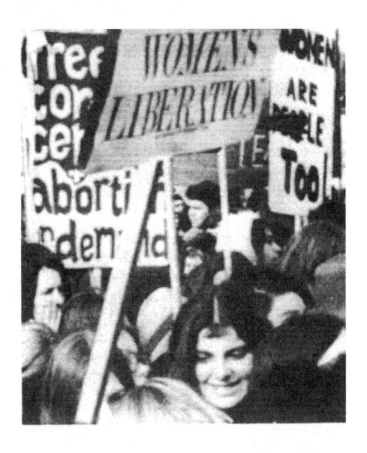

But it would be naive to assume that, because all women experience medical sexism, all women have the same needs and priorities at this time. Class differences in the medical treatment of women may not be as sharp as they were eighty years ago, but they are still very real. For black women, medical racism often overshadows medical sexism. For poor women of all ethnic groups, the problem of how to get services of any kind often overshadows all qualitative concerns. And for all of us except the most affluent, there is the constant worry about whether the care we are getting meets minimal standards of technical competence—never mind the amenities of dignity and courtesy.

A movement that recognizes our biological similarity but denies the diversity of our priorities cannot be a women's health movement, it can only be *some women's* health movement. For example, it is important to demand a more dignified and participatory approach to childbirth. But to focus on the demand that we be allowed to experience the beauty of childbirth—while thousands of women do not have adequate prenatal nutrition, or have not had access to the means of avoiding unwanted childbearing—is worse than naive: it is cruel.

It is easy enough to say that we must recognize the diversity of women's needs, and that the demands we make of the medical system must represent the broadest possible range of women's experience. But once we begin to talk about needs beyond the most minimal survival services (contraception, cancer screening, etc.), we are no longer on very firm ground. How much of our "need" is manufactured, and how much is real?

For example, the medical handling of pregnancy in our culture undoubtedly contributes to our anxieties about pregnancy, and anxiety can transform a minor discomfort into an urgent *need* for medical attention. The "need" is real enough at the time, but in a sense it is artificial, manufactured to enhance our dependency on the medical system. Or, more commonly, our very ignorance of our bodies sometimes sends us in search of information and reassurance when no real care is necessary—another case of manufactured dependency.

On the other hand, for all our anger at being dismissed as "psychosomatic" cases when we really do feel sick, we cannot rule out the possibility that many women use sickness as an escape from their oppression as workers and wives. They are not being dishonest, or faking. Our culture encourages people to express resistance as "illness," just as it encourages us to view overt rebellion as "sick." The oppression is real; the resistance is real; but the sickness is manufactured.

Just how "sick" are we then as women? How much of our dependence on the medical system is biological necessity, and how much is social artifice? We spoke before of the contradiction between our rejection of medical ideology and our real dependence on medical technology. But how much of that dependency *is* real?

Have we been so blinded by the ideology (which labels us sick, one way or another) that we cannot define the dependency?

The women's movement has been totally ambivalent about this issue. There are feminists who would deny that we have any special liabilities as women: to them menstrual cramps, nausea in pregnancy, and all the rest are culturally induced, "curable" with a dose of consciousness-raising and a short course in physiology. However, there are other feminists who seem totally preoccupied with the agonies of menstruation, postpartum depression, or menopause. And there are some who believe that childbirth is so dangerous and so degrading that we should abstain until test-tube babies are available. And there are feminists who believe that childbirth is so healthy and gratifying that it is the peak experience of a woman's life. We seem to alternate between accusing the medical system of treating us as if we were sick and accusing them of not appreciating how sick we are!

The trouble is that whatever we say can be, and is, used against us. Say that menstruation is painful and distressing, and women will be arbitrarily barred from occupations that involve concentration and responsibility. Say that it is unnoticeable and that we are as consistently healthy as males are supposed to be, and all women will be required to lift the same weights and work the same long hours required of men regardless of the degree of discomfort experienced. Say that the last months of pregnancy are difficult, and we will be fired at the first signs of swelling. Say that there is "nothing unhealthy about being pregnant," and we will be held to eight hours a day, five days a week. There are real dangers—for all of us—in either understating or exaggerating our needs as women.

There is no "correct line" on our bodies. There is no way to determine our "real" needs, our "real" strengths and liabilities, in a sexist society—any more than there is a way to understand what "female nature" may really be. How can we "know ourselves" when the only images we have of ourselves are images cast by an oppressive society?

There is no way for us to come to terms with our own bodies, in whatever female "subcultures" we may attempt to create, because, when you come right down to it, our *bodies* are not the issue. Biology is not the issue. The issue is power, in all the ways it affects us. We could debate endlessly, for example, about whether premenstrual tension is "real" or psychosomatic, whether the last months of pregnancy are invigorating or debilitating. But the real question is: Who decides the consequences? We could clash over the

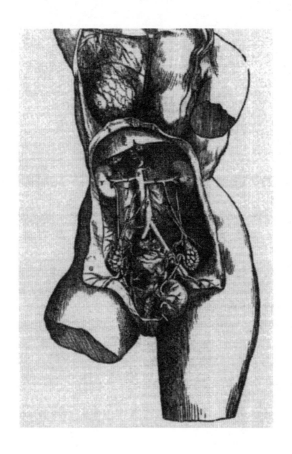

culture of childbirth, whether or not having test-tube babies would be "healthier" and more liberating than natural childbirth. But who decides what options will actually be available to us? More important, who controls the social context of childbirth—the availability of abortion at one end and of day care at the other?

This is not to say that we do not need more hard information about our biology and about our health needs. We do. We need to know much more about occupational health hazards specific to women, about actual emotional patterns accompanying menstruation and pregnancy, about the potential hazards of various contraceptive methods, and about many other areas ignored or distorted by medicine. But in our concern to understand more about our own biology, for our own purposes, we must never lose sight of the fact that it is not our *biology* that oppresses us—but a social system based on sex and class domination.

This, to us, is the most profoundly liberating feminist insight—the understanding that our oppression is socially, and not biologically, ordained. To act on this understanding is to ask for more than "control over our own bodies." It is to ask for, and struggle for, control over the social options available to us, and control over all the institutions of society that now define those options.

Bibliography

[As appeared in the original 1973 printing.]

I.

For more perspective on medical sexism in contemporary society, you should read:

Chesler, Phyllis. *Women and Madness*. New York: Doubleday, 1972. On sexist theory and practice in psychiatry. A best seller for good reasons.

Frankfort, Ellen. *Vaginal Politics*. New York: Quadrangle Books, 1972. Wide-ranging, lucid report on medical sexism today from abortion to cancer and sexuality.

Lennane, K. Jean, and R. John Lennane. "Alleged Psychogenic Disorders in Women – A Possible Manifestation of Sexual Prejudice." In *New England Journal of Medicine* 288 (1973): 288. Two doctors attack the medical profession's tendency to diagnose women's illness as psychosomatic.

Scully, Diane, and Bart, Pauline. "A Funny Thing Happened on the Way to the Orifice: Women in Gynecology Textbooks." In *American Journal of Sociology* 78 (1973): 1045. Long overdue feminist study of the textbooks gynecologists read and write.

Seaman, Barbara. *Free and Female.* New York: Coward-McCann, 1972. See especially the chapter on gynecologists. Fun to read and full of information.

Szasz, Thomas S. *The Myth of Mental Illness.* New York: Dell, 1961. Psychiatry exposed as an agency of social control. A classic.

II.

If you want to read more about the history, these are some of the sources we found especially useful, for their interpretations as well as for their information:

Barker-Benfield, Ben. "The Spermatic Economy: A Nineteenth Century View of Sexuality." In *Feminist Studies* 1, no. 1 (Summer 1972). Fascinating study of male motivation in gynecology and the relationship between medical ideas and the

economic basis of society—by a truly feminist
male historian.

Cott, Nancy F., ed. *Root of Bitterness: Documents of
the Social History of American Women.* New York:
Dutton, 1972. See especially the section, "Sexuality and Gynecology in the Nineteenth Century."

Fruchter, Rachel Gillett. "Women's Weakness: Consumption and Women in the Nineteenth Century."
Unpublished paper, 1973. The source of all our
information on women and TB.

Gilman, Charlotte Perkins. *The Yellow Wall-Paper.*
With an afterword by Elaine R. Hedges. Old
Westbury, New York: The Feminist Press, 1973.
Great as literature as well as being a socially pen-
etrating description of female invalidism.

Higham, John. *Strangers in the Land: Patterns of
American Nativism (1860–1925).* New York: Ath-
eneum, 1971. The chapter on the development of
racism is full of insight into the ideological uses
of "science."

Kennedy, David M. *Birth Control in America: The
Career of Margaret Sanger.* New Haven: Yale
University Press, 1970. Excellent as a biography
and a social history. Shows (with a minimum of
sexism) why Margaret Sanger was not a radical
or a feminist.

Pivar, David J. *The New Abolitionism: The Quest for Social Purity (1876–1900)*. Ann Arbor: University Microfilms, 1965. Traces the antislavery movement up to later social reform movements spearheaded by middle- and upper-class women. A valuable source for us.

Rosenberg, Charles E. *The Cholera Years*. Chicago and London: The University of Chicago Press, 1962. The only public health history we know of that puts public health in historical and social perspective. A key source to us.

Smith-Rosenberg, Carroll. "The Hysterical Woman: Sex Roles in Nineteenth Century America." In *Social Research* 39, no. 4 (Winter 1972): 652–78. An excellent article that focuses on the doctor-patient relationship.

Vicinus, Martha, ed. *Suffer and Be Still: Women in the Victorian Age*. Bloomington and London: Indiana University Press, 1972. A scholarly anthology ranging from menstruation to women in art.

Zaretsky, Eli. "Capitalism, the Family and Personal Life." In *Socialist Revolution* 3, nos. 13 and 14 (January–April 1973): 69–125. Sweeping historical analysis of the relationship between women's roles and the economic system.

If you want to do further research, you might want to look at some of the following books and articles. Some are widely available; others are obscure. (We used the New York Academy of Medicine Library and the main branch of the New York Public Library at Forty-Second Street and Fifth Avenue):

General Social History

Banks, J. A., and Banks, Olive. *Feminism and Family Planning in Victorian England.* New York: Schocken Books, 1964. Really much broader than the title suggests. Describes the development of the "lady" and her social role.

Crow, Duncan. *The Victorian Woman.* New York: Stein and Day, 1971. Wide-ranging and fun to read. The emphasis is on English women.

Hofstadter, Richard. *The Age of Reform.* New York: Alfred A. Knopf, 1965.

Mann, Arthur. *Yankee Reformers in the Urban Age.* Cambridge, Massachusetts: Belknap Press, 1954.

The above books by Hofstadter and Mann provide some general historical background on urban life and politics in the late nineteenth and early twentieth centuries.

Histories of Medicine, Public Health, and Disease

Graham, Harvey. *Eternal Eve: The Mystery of Birth and the Customs That Surround It.* London: Hutchinson and Co., 1960. A totally uncritical history of gynecology and obstetrics.

Freud, Sigmund. *Dora—An Analysis of a Case of Hysteria.* New York: Collier Books, 1963. The discovery that hysteria was a mental disorder; the beginning of psychoanalysis.

Rosebury, Theodor. *Microbes and Morals: The Strange Story of Venereal Disease.* New York: Ballantine Books, 1971. Explores the (sometimes sexist) myths surrounding VD.

Rosen, George. *A History of Public Health.* New York: MD Publications, 1958. Like most public health histories, this one focuses on the march of science and gives very little sociological interpretation.

Szasz, Thomas S. "The Sane Slave: An Historical Note on the Use of Medical Diagnosis as Justificatory Rhetoric." In *American Journal of Psychotherapy* 25, no. 2 (April 1971): 228–39. A discussion of Dr. Samuel Cartwright's medical theories about blacks.

Veith, Ilza. *Hysteria: The History of A Disease.* Chicago and London: The University of Chicago Press, 1965. A rich and detailed history.

Winslow, C. E. A. *The Evolution and Significance of the Modern Public Health Campaign*. New Haven: Yale University Press, 1923. A leading historian of public health considers the relationship of public health measures to scientific advance—nothing on public health and society.

Nineteenth-Century Medical Books on Women

Bliss, W. W. *Woman, and Her Thirty-Years' Pilgrimage*. Boston: B. B. Russell, 1870.

Clarke, Edward H., MD. *Sex in Education, or, a Fair Chance for the Girls*. Boston: James R. Osgood and Co., 1873. Reprint Edition 1972 by Arno Press, Inc. The famous diatribe against higher education for women.

Dirix, M. E., MD. *Woman's Complete Guide to Health*. New York: W. A. Townsend and Adams, 1869.

Hollick, F., MD. *The Diseases of Woman, Their Cause and Cure Familiarly Explained*. New York: T.W. Strong, 1849.

Taylor, W. C., MD. *A Physician's Counsels to Woman in Health and Disease*. Springfield: W. J. Holland & Co., 1871.

Warner, Lucien C., MD. *A Popular Treatise on the Functions and Diseases of Woman*. New York: Manhattan Publishing Company, 1874.

Home Economics and Sanitation

Campbell, Helen. *Household Economics.* New York:
G. P. Putnam's Sons, 1907. Post-germ theory
treatise on the "science" of housekeeping.

Plunkett, H. M., Mrs. *Women, Plumbers and Doctors, or
Household Sanitation.* New York: Appleton, 1885.
Spells out the woman's responsibility as sanitation officer in her own home, filled with fears of
contagion from the poor.

Wright, Julia McNair. *The Complete Home: An Encyclo-
pedia of Domestic Life and Affairs.* Philadelphia:
P. W. Ziegler and Co., 1881. Wherein "Aunt Soph-
ronia" advises her nieces on how to manage the
house (i.e., the servants).

Birth Control

Complete Works of Theodore Roosevelt. Vol. 19. New
York: Charles Scribner's Sons, 1926. See Chapter
Twelve, "Birth Reform from the Positive, Not the
Negative Side," pp. 152–66.

Sanger, Margaret. *Woman and the New Race.* New
York: Brentano's Publishing Co., 1920. Blames
motherhood for all human misery and pins the
survival of "the race" (the human race minus the
"unfit") on birth control.

Miscellaneous

Reverby, Susan. *Sex O'Clock in America: Prostitution, White Slavery, the Progressives and the Jews (1900–1917)*. Unpublished, 1973. Anti-Semitism in the antivice movement, and much more.

Salmon, Lucy Maynard. *Domestic Service.* New York: Macmillan, 1911. The definitive historical and statistical study of servants in America. The dry facts are enlivened with a wealth of quotes from servants and mistresses.

Soper, George A. "The Curious Career of Typhoid Mary." In the magazine *The Diplomate* (December 1939). The story of her capture, by the man who captured her.

Walker, Stanley. "Typhoid Carrier #36." In *The New Yorker,* January 26, 1935. A sympathetic account of Typhoid Mary's last years on North Brother Island.

Woolston, Howard B. *Prostitution in the U.S.* New Jersey: Patterson Smith Reprint Series, 1969 (copyright 1921). Part of the Rockefeller-sponsored series on vice. The statistics are probably sound, but the interpretations are frequently outrageous.

Education Department of the ILGWU, New York. *Garment Workers Speak.* The horrors of early twentieth-century factory work—by the women who survived.

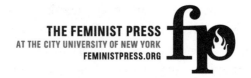